the
Stutterer's
Survival
guide

NICHOLAS
TUNBRIDGE

Addison-Wesley Publishing Company

Sydney • Wokingham, England • Reading, Massachusetts
Menlo Park, California • New York • Don Mills, Ontario
Amsterdam • Bonn • Singapore • Tokyo • Madrid
San Juan • Mexico City • Paris • Milan • Seoul

To anybody who has ever had to deal with stuttering and to my wife, Astrid, for her never-ending love and support.

Acquisitions Editor: Wendy Rapee
Production Editor: Susan Lewis
Copy Editor: Shirley Jones
Text and cover design by Carol Hudson
Illustrations by Mike Spoor
Author photograph by Ron Rapee

Typeset by DOCUPRO, Sydney
Printed in Australia by McPherson's Printing Group

National Library of Australia
Cataloguing-in-Publication

Tunbridge, Nicholas.
  The stutterer's survival guide.

  ISBN 0 201 44356 2.

  1. Stuttering—Treatment. 2. Self-care, Health. I. Title.
616.855406

CONTENTS

FOREWORD   vii

CHAPTER ONE
SO YOU ARE A ST . . . ST . . . STUTTERER   1

    GROWING UP WITH A STUTTER   2
    OVERCOMING A STUTTER   4

CHAPTER TWO
TECHNIQUES THAT WORK FOR ME   7

    THE PROBLEM ELEMENTS   9
      Speed   9
      Thinking before you speak   11
    A WORD ON TECHNIQUES   12
      Crawl with the technique   13
      Learning to use technique   14
    THE SPEECH DIARY   15

CHAPTER THREE
DESENSITISING: GETTING OVER THE EMBARRASSMENT   19

    WHAT IS DESENSITISATION?   20
      On the trail of fluency   21
      Overcoming self-consciousness   22
    HOW TO DESENSITISE YOURSELF   26
      Voluntary stuttering   26
      Slowing down   27
      Do not be self-conscious   28
    LOOKING AT THE 'WHY' OF STUTTERING   31
      The stuttering loop   33

TACKLING DIFFICULT SITUATIONS   **35**
    Replacing negative feelings with positive feelings   **38**

CHAPTER FOUR
STARVING THE STUTTER   **41**

    FOUR TABOOS   **42**
        Word avoidance   **43**
        Situation avoidance   **48**
        Spontaneous fluency   **51**
        Filler sounds   **53**
    OVERCOMPENSATING AT WORK   **54**

CHAPTER FIVE
YOU AND YOUR SPEECH BUDDIES   **58**

    WHAT YOU NEED FROM SPEECH BUDDIES   **60**
    THE IMPORTANCE OF PRACTICE   **62**
        Daily practice   **62**
        A hierarchy of assignments   **65**

CHAPTER SIX
FAMILY, FRIENDS AND OTHERS   **75**

    FAMILY AND FRIENDS   **76**
        Speaking with family and friends   **79**
    PEOPLE'S REACTIONS TO STUTTERERS   **80**
        Put yourself in the stutterer's shoes   **82**
    IF YOUR CHILD STUTTERS   **83**

CHAPTER SEVEN
HOT SPOTS   **86**

    SCHOOLDAYS   **87**
        Answering questions   **88**
        Asking questions   **91**

CONTENTS

Reading aloud   91
Giving a presentation   92
Parties   93
Enjoying your schooldays   94
AT WORK   95
Making introductions   95
Speaking at a meeting   98
The interview   100
The important phone call   103
The presentation   109
Client meeting with colleague/manager   112
IMPORTANT SOCIAL MOMENTS   113
COPING WITH STRESS, ILLNESS AND FATIGUE   116
Coping with stress   116
Coping with illness   117
Coping with fatigue   119
Coping with those stuttery days   120
Coping with difficult people   123
A FINAL WORD ON HOT SPOTS   125

CHAPTER EIGHT
WHERE DO WE GO FROM HERE?   126

WHEN THINGS GO WRONG   127
AN ATTAINABLE DREAM   128

FINAL TIPS FOR YOUR SURVIVAL KIT   131

FOREWORD

We know a lot about stuttering. In childhood it affects five people in every one hundred. We aren't sure of the exact rate of stuttering among adults but one in two hundred is probably a conservative estimate. Three times as many boys stutter than do girls, and this disproportion increases with age. This means that among adults who stutter we find many more men than women.

While most studies of stuttering have been based in western countries, we know that the characteristic repetitions, prolongations and blocking of sounds have been observed to impede the smooth flow of speech in speakers right throughout the world. Wherever it has been sought, stuttering has been found in every language and among members of every race. It knows no societal or characterological barriers. It exists among the rich and the poor, the educated and the naive, the sophisticated and the primitive. Likewise it is found among the bold and the timid, the placid and the anxious, the gregarious and the retiring.

Stuttering is not an emotional disorder. People who stutter, and for that matter their parents, have no greater tendency to be anxious or neurotic than the rest of the population. While psychological factors can influence the course of the disorder, the basic problem is a physical one. People who stutter do so because the complex part of the brain that controls the muscles we use to speak does not work as efficiently as it should in all circumstances.

It's well known that stuttering runs in families and it was often suggested that the disorder was 'learned' or environmentally generated. We now know that the disorder is largely inherited, with genetic factors more than twice as influential as environmental ones.

Having a stutter is a bit like driving on ice when you're inexperienced. You know where you want to go and you try to make the car go there but it's easy to skid into disaster. Even if you do manage to stay on your chosen path, control is tenuous and you never quite know when you'll lose it. The more demanding the situation, the harder it is to maintain the control you have. So, if it's slippery and you're worrying about the appointment you're going to, or your passenger is being argumentative, or you're tired and cold, you're much more vulnerable to accident than in easier circumstances.

It is the same for stuttering. Your brain doesn't have good, reliable control over the complex co-ordinated muscular movements that produce speech. When things are going comfortably, when you're at ease with your listener and saying something simple and straightforward, you're much more likely to be fluent than if you're talking on a difficult topic to an unfamiliar audience or when you're asking the boss for a raise. These demanding situations divert 'brain power' away from your speech control and your fluency breaks down.

Most people who stutter first do so in early childhood. For some the problem goes away during the natural course of maturation of the nervous system. Often the disfluency comes at a time when language acquisition or communication demands are outstripping the development of adequate speech control. When this catches up, the stuttering resolves. But for others this doesn't happen, or it happens too late. The longer the stutter persists, the less likely it is to remit naturally, and those still stuttering beyond puberty face a lifetime of chronic disfluency unless treatment intervenes.

These days we don't wait to see which path a child's stuttering will take. If you are concerned that your child is abnormally disfluent, especially if there is a family history of stuttering, you should seek a professional assessment immediately, even if the child is only pre-school age. Early treatment is important as it allows changes to be made at a time when the nervous system is most flexible.

If you're reading this as someone who has reached adulthood with a stutter, you may feel that you've missed the boat. This is definitely not the case because excellent adult treatment is available. Granted, it's much harder work than in childhood, a little like 'teaching an old dog new tricks' but, unlike in the proverb, it *can* be done.

Even a long lifetime of stuttering is no bar to gaining reliably fluent speech if you are willing to work hard at your therapy and to carry that commitment on into your everyday life. The strategy of maintaining your hard won fluency after treatment is what this valuable little book is all about. If you've already been through treatment you'll be keen to move on to that message. If you haven't, you'll want to know what treatment entails.

There's no magic in treatment. You can't go along to a therapist, be given the secret of fluency and leave cured. And it's not like having a pacemaker put in or a gallstone taken out, where the surgeon does something clever and you walk away with the problem solved. While we're now sure we're dealing with a physical problem, it isn't one for which there is a satisfactory physical treatment.

In rare circumstances there are people whose stuttering is associated with another problem, like a head injury, and here surgery or medication may have a role, but in general this isn't the case.

We know there are physical interventions which have given some people who stutter temporary improvement in fluency, and these include certain powerful drugs, muscle relaxants and various electronic devices which alter the way the speaker hears himself. Unfortunately these tend to be fraught with unacceptable side effects or inconvenience, and nothing along this line has yet proved effective as a long-term treatment.

When you undertake good treatment for stuttering you have to be active, not passive. You have to put the treatment into practice yourself, getting your brain to do things it finds hard. It isn't something that someone or something does to you. It is this sort of treatment that this book presumes you've tackled.

Good treatment means first learning a skill. To refer back to the analogy of driving on ice, good treatment teaches you how to become a reliable driver despite the unfavourable conditions. The exact technique that you learn varies with the treatment program that you enter, but skill in dealing with your inefficient speech control system is the important first step.

Whatever technique you learn, it's also important that it's one which allows good, natural sounding speech when you've mastered it. Singing is usually a quick way to produce fluency but it isn't any use as a treatment unless you want to go around sounding like a Gilbert and Sullivan operetta. If you don't like the way you sound after therapy you're unlikely to get any lasting benefit.

Initially you learn your new skills in the safe environment of a clinic. In terms of our analogy it's like learning to drive on a simulator. Then gradually you move what you have learned into the real world, without much traffic at first, slowly building up to greater challenges.

Skill isn't the only component of good treatment. You also have to convince yourself that the skill will see you through even the most formidable situations. It's no use being the racing driver who can get around the empty track better than everyone else if you can't win the actual race. So it's also important for treatment to help you deal with things that hold you back in proving yourself. Such comprehensive treatment is known as cognitive behavioural therapy and its effectiveness in stuttering is well established.

Of course to undertake this sort of treatment, which is often offered intensively, you have to be prepared to invest real time and effort, which means you have to be highly motivated to make a change in your fluency. And, more than that, you have to stay motivated if you want a good long-term result. If you don't use the skills you've learned, you'll lose them. You can't keep them packed up in a carrybag like a Superman suit that you can jump into when danger looms. People have done that, only to find that the suit gets progressively moth-eaten until it's no good at all. You also can't afford to start avoiding old difficulties because they'll quickly resume their former status. You have to have the courage and conviction to take what you have learned in treatment and use it consistently in your everyday life.

You can have the best therapist in the world, just as you can have the best coach, the best maestro, the best guide, but in the end it's you who has to win the game, play the concerto, climb the mountain. Similarly, with gaining and keeping reliable fluency, it's you who does the talking. And, more than that, its you and only you who takes the ultimate responsibility for success, along with the credit that accompanies it.

This book tells you how one very successful person has tackled that responsibility. It tells you about the process of becoming your own therapist, the ultimate goal of good treatment.

Nick Tunbridge practises what he preaches. I can assure you that if you were to meet Nick today and didn't know his story, you'd be unlikely to notice anything at all unusual about the way he talks, other than that he's a fine speaker who communicates exceptionally well. As you'll learn from the pages of this book, this mastery is hard won but the important message is — it is most definitely winnable.

Megan Neilson PhD
Director of the Stuttering Treatment Program
CRUfAD, University of New South Wales at
St Vincent's Hospital

CHAPTER ONE

SO YOU ARE A ST . . . ST . . . STUTTERER

This guide is written by a stutterer for other stutterers. Every stutterer meets little disasters and emotional catastrophes every day that only other stutterers can fully appreciate. I have taught myself how to handle both the ordinary and the difficult situation without stuttering and my quality of life has significantly improved as a result. I feel that, through this book, I can help you too.

The Stutterer's Survival Guide aims to get the stutterer through each day. It outlines steps you can take to maintain your fluency and dignity and it also provides some advice on handling those speech 'hot spots' that arise from time to time.

This is not a technical or scientific manual, nor does it in any way attempt to replace the role of the therapist. My sole claim to expertise is that I have stuttered for most of my life and have been through most therapy programs in an attempt to stop stuttering. I know what stutterers go through.

I believe that being able to pull a 'speech companion' out of your pocket to consult when things get difficult — a speech companion that offers constructive advice and supports you in your quest for fluency — would be of great help to the stutterer. This guide is, I believe, just such a companion.

GROWING UP WITH A STUTTER

All parents hope and pray that their new-born baby will be healthy, normal and live a happy and full life. There I was, a healthy, happy baby and a 'normal' healthy kid until I was about five. Then an interesting transformation took place — I started to show signs that when I spoke I was not like all the other kids. I stuttered. Everyone assumed I'd just grow out of it.

By the time I was ten, I was bigger and stronger, and guess what? My stutter had gotten bigger and stronger right there along with the rest of me! I was aware I had trouble speaking sometimes, but I did not know what all the fuss was about. My friends didn't mind. Nobody seemed to mind except the teacher and mum and dad. I remember very clearly my mother driving me every Friday afternoon to see a speech therapist who lived in the city. I would spend an hour playing with toys while the therapist 'talked' to my mother. I do not think this helped my mother much and it was certainly little help to me.

By the time I was in my teens I was even taller and stronger, and I really liked girls and motorbikes, but I didn't feel I was enjoying myself like everyone else. My stutter seemed here to stay. Sometimes I could feel my friends getting embarrassed when I had problems with my speech and sometimes they would laugh. Calling a girl up on the phone for a date was much harder for me than for the rest of the guys, because I couldn't say the words I wanted to. The girl would say hello over and over again, and then hang up. I would be left sweating and shaking.

I began to realise that I was having a really hard time talking. And that really worried me. Talking was something all of us have to do over and over every day — and it wasn't getting any easier for me. Not only was I having to go through all the mixed up and confused emotions that all young people go through, but I was also having to cope with the fact that I stuttered and could not speak without becoming embarrassed. Imagine what it is like for a 17 year old who is trying to act cool to find he can't even say his own name without tripping up on it.

Stutterers get through their adolescence as best as they can. By the time they get to their early twenties they have developed their own system for survival to get them through their life.

The work place can be lonely because not many stutterers end up working with other stutterers.

If you are a stutterer with problems at home, at school or at work, this guide will not only make you realise that you are not alone, but will also offer you some constructive advice to enable you to get through each day a little more easily.

OVERCOMING A STUTTER

Let's take stock of ourselves. We are perfectly normal, happy individuals — until we have to speak. As soon as we try to come out with something, people look puzzled or horrified as if we have grown a second head. Or they shrink away from us. You know the scene? It happens to all stutterers.

Let's look at it from the other side. If you were a 'normal' fluent speaker who had never before met anyone who stuttered, how would you react? You would probably experience one or perhaps several of these feelings:

- Embarrassment
- Pity
- Anger
- Amusement.

These are absolutely normal reactions. You have to accept the fact that when you stutter your speech sounds strange and to some people it can be very funny. This may seem cruel, but it is a fact. I would suggest to you at this very early point of our journey together that you accept the following statements:

- You have a stutter
- You sound rather strange when you stutter
- Different people have different reactions to stutterers.

If, magically, you had the chance to change one thing in your life what would it be? In most cases the one thing a stutterer would like is to get rid of their stutter. Well, believe it or not, you *can* stop stuttering. I have done it and I know of others that, by following certain rules, have been successful as well.

First, though, you have to accept the fact that you have a stutter and that it is affecting your quality of life. I believe any stutterer offered the chance to become fluent would take it, even if it meant downing a witch's brew or following instant remedies based on old wives tales such as, 'If you stand upside down, balance two lead weights on your feet and count from 1000 backwards, you will stop stuttering!'. Two words of good advice about all instant remedies for stuttering — forget them!

I know of people who have tried everything, who have travelled the world searching for a cure — and they still stutter. To the stutterer, stuttering is normal; speaking fluently is not. To overcome your stutter, you will have to go right back to the beginning and change something that you have been doing naturally for most of your life. That will not happen overnight. The attitude I want you to acquire is that fluency is something you have to work on every minute of the day. Attaining fluency will eventually become relatively easy, but you have a history of stuttering to overcome.

If you are anything like me, particular words, syllables and situations always give trouble. When you head into these 'hot spots', your mind is screaming at you 'This is a stutter zone — get ready to stutter!!' and what happens? Instant block. It is going to take time and effort to rewrite that message with something positive, but it can be done.

In the next chapter I'll describe what I do.

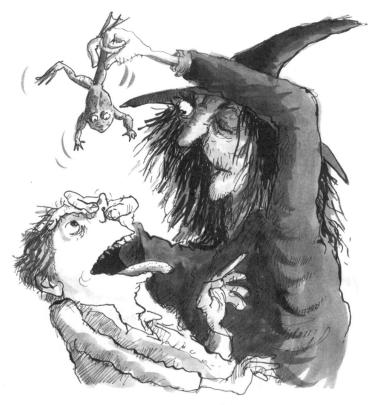

CHAPTER TWO

TECHNIQUES
THAT
WORK
FOR ME

This guide is not designed to teach you a speech technique to stop stuttering. What I describe in this guide is what I do to maintain my fluency (and stay sane) after having been through years of therapy. My intensive therapy ended after I learned what is called the 'fluency shaping method'. The therapy may have ended, but the practical work started and will never end. I will spend a little time on some elements of that technique, which I feel are of universal benefit. Remember though, that a technique that works for me may not work for someone else.

I am assuming that you, as a stutterer, have some kind of technique or system to get you through the day. Whether you have a technique or not, you should read this guide. It is going to help you to some degree in some way. If you want to know more about techniques, I suggest you see a speech therapist, learn a technique then read this guide again.

Let's recap. You have a technique. Perhaps it's not working or not working as well as you would like; or perhaps it works well, until certain situations arise. This guide gives straightforward descriptions of what I do to overcome problems. I also give specific examples of what I consider difficult situations and outline strategies to remove or at the least minimise the problems associated with them.

As I said earlier, I have chosen two elements that I consider to be of benefit no matter what your technique. These two elements are *speed* and *thinking before you speak*. Does this sound simple? Yes, it does, but not many speakers, fluent or otherwise, practise them.

THE PROBLEM ELEMENTS

■ SPEED

YOU ARE ALWAYS ON PROBATION

When you pass your driving licence test in Australia you are given a probationary licence and you are required to display a 'P' plate on the front and rear of the vehicle. After 12 months, if you haven't been caught breaking any regulations, you are awarded a full licence and can remove the 'P' plates. The 'P' plates are required so that other drivers are aware that you are a probationary driver and therefore do not possess the same level of experience and skill as other drivers. The 'P' plater is also restricted to travelling at a slower speed than full licence holders.

I want you to imagine that you have a 'P' plate attached to you. You are a probationary 'fluent speaker' and you are certainly restricted by the speed that you can speak. When you hear other speakers 'racing' along, remember that they have a 'full' licence. It is probably a good idea to consider yourself on probation from this day on. Although things will get easier for you, you will always remain, even though you may have stopped stuttering, a probationary speaker.

Speech, like walking or running, can be measured by speed. With running or walking we measure the speed in kilometres per hour; speech we measure in syllables per minute (spm). Most fluent speakers speak somewhere around 200–280 spm. People who speak very quickly are speaking at around the 280 spm mark. Slow speakers are probably speaking at around 180–200 spm. When you are not stuttering, you are probably speaking at around 240 to 270 spm. To measure your speed, just count how many syllables you are speaking in a 20-second period and multiply it by three. This tells you how many syllables you are speaking on average per minute.

I would guess that you are probably speaking at a speed that's too fast for you to handle. It's like trying to drive an old car at the same speed as a new sports car. You will lose control and eventually crash.

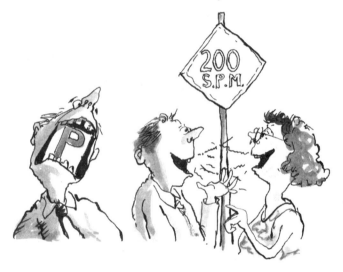

My speech rate used to be 275 spm. I now speak at 200–220 spm. I try to keep my speed down to 200, or even lower. If I speed up to 220 I know that I am too close to my limit and run the risk of stuttering.

Different people normally speak at different rates. Some are quite comfortable speaking at 180 spm, some are comfortable at 300 spm. If you are a stutterer, you will have a much higher chance of maintaining fluency if you slow your speech rate down. I would suggest that you aim for 200 spm.

Measure and monitor your speech rate regularly. Aim for 200 syllables per minute, which may possibly be somewhere around 70% of your current speed.

■ THINKING BEFORE YOU SPEAK

How often do you really think about what you are going to say before you say it? I'm not talking about the millisecond between the thought and the sound. I'm talking about carefully thinking out what you are going to say before you say it. If you are anything like I used to be you probably do not give it much thought at all.

Imagine, if you can, that you have a huge screen in front of you at all times, so close that you can see it, feel it, smell it, touch it. Everything you are going to say is printed on that screen. There are three main advantages in using an imaginary screen.

- Firstly, you will speak more slowly. The process between thinking what you are going to say and speaking those thoughts will be automatically slowed, because you have introduced a visual component (your screen) into the process.
- Secondly, you will have additional time to get your speech in order. By this I mean that you will have time to consciously ensure that your technique is in place and this will reduce the likelihood of bursts of 'spontaneous' fluency which can lead to speech 'dead ends'.
- Thirdly, you get to keep your friends. Believe me, it's impossible to put your foot in your mouth if you use this imaginary screen.

Did you get the message? I'll repeat it once again.
■ Firstly, slow down.
■ Secondly, think out what you want to say before you say it.

A WORD ON TECHNIQUES

When I refer to 'technique' throughout this book, I refer to techniques that you as a stutterer use to enable you to speak as fluently as possible. You may have learned these techniques in a clinic, quite possibly from professionals such as speech pathologists. Alternatively, you may have developed your own technique, one that works well for you.

According to my investigations there are two main 'clinic' techniques. These are:
■ the fluency shaping technique which I have studied, and now practise; and
■ the stuttering modification technique.
The fluency shaping technique teaches you to become fluent by linking the sounds together and by concentrating on breathing, phrasing and pausing. The stuttering modification technique promotes fluency by controlled stuttering.

A word of warning on 'homemade' techniques. They may or may not be valid. Be very careful that you have not refined word avoidance or situation avoidance to such an extent that you have come up with some kind of behavioural modification that you label as your 'technique'. (See Chapter 4 for a detailed discussion of word avoidance and situation avoidance.) It may be that every time you feel tension you inhale a great amount of air, or you speak very loudly, or cough or, as I have seen in some cases, stamp your foot.

The aim of a technique should be to give you fluent speech in a practical and normal way. In other words, by using your technique you should be able to say what you want, when you want to say it, and not be a spectacle. If your technique does not enable you to do that, I would consider it not a fluency enhancing technique, but an 'avoidance'-based technique. If you want to improve your 'homemade' technique, I suggest you contact a speech clinic and discuss the situation with professionals. Find out about the various techniques available and by all means ask them to evaluate yours. You never know, you may be giving the speech professionals valuable information that may help them in their research.

■ CRAWL WITH THE TECHNIQUE

I am assuming that you have already undertaken treatment at a clinic. You will have had, at the best, a total of three weeks use of your technique. You have been given the absolute basics. Comparing this with driving a car, you know how to open the door and start the motor, and that's about it. So do not go racing. Learn to drive first.

You now have to learn how to use the technique and use it so that it fits your lifestyle. You have to become an expert in its use. This is your way out of stuttering. You have to know how your technique relates to you and what you can and cannot do with it. Stretch it to the limit. Try it in all kinds of situations. Become obsessed by it. You have to use this new way of speaking every time you open your mouth. You have to know what situations will require more, what situations will require less use of technique. You have to know how far you can stretch it, and how fast you can speak.

Live, breath, think and dream your technique. It's your way out of the stuttering jungle.

■ LEARNING TO USE TECHNIQUE

After you have finished treatment, your main emphasis must be on daily practice. I suggest at least two sessions of 30 minutes a day for the first few months, if you can fit them into your schedule. If you cannot, then change your priorities to fit them in. If you are really serious about stopping stuttering, I do not think spending one hour a day for the first few months is unreasonable to improve the quality of your life by 100%, do you?

RECORDING YOUR SPEECH

One of the most useful tools to assist you in the monitoring and evaluation of your speech is the pocket tape-recorder or dictaphone. I use a voice-activated one that I carry in the inside pocket of my jacket. Because the tape-recorder is very close to you, it picks up *your* speech, but not the speech of those around you. This, however, is what you want. You are using it to evaluate how *you speak*, not to record the conversation.

A tape-recording of your speech, particularly in a stressful situation, gives you the most accurate and honest report of how you are speaking. There is an additional benefit in using a tape-recorder. Just having it with you and feeling the weight of it in your pocket serves as a reminder to you to use your technique.

After you have finished your taping session, evaluate your speech. You should monitor your speech regularly. *Note: In Australia, it is illegal to tape-record a conversation without the agreement of all parties.*

The speech diary

After your treatment you will realise that you have a long journey in front of you. This journey will be full of obstacles. You will have the occasional problem and hopefully more than the occasional success. A good idea is to keep a speech diary so that you can record your speech throughout your speaking day. This will provide you with a record of how you 'travelled' after learning your technique. If you write in it daily it also helps to keep you focused on your speech and in particular brings to your attention any trouble spots that you may need to deal with.

It can be useful to record your speech experiences in a diary. When you have a bad day, make a comment about why you thought you had the problem and what you intend to do about it next time. Talk it over with your friends who stutter, that is, your 'speech buddies' (see Chapter 5). Ask their opinion of why they thought you had the problem and see if they agree with your thoughts as to how to avoid the problem in the future.

I have included some excerpts from my diary to give you an idea of the sort of daily speech events that I considered important to note. One great benefit of keeping a speech diary is that you can go back and see how much you have improved. Even today when I go back over my diary I am amazed at how much trouble I had in the beginning. It really is worth the couple of minutes it takes every night to write it up.

One last thing, don't just record bad news in your diary, make a point of writing down something good about your speech every day.

Tuesday, 5 April
Today's Goal: Speech rate 180 spm

Practice Session — morning
30 minutes with speech buddy. Majority of practice done at 180 spm, my 'target' speed for the day. Speech buddy and I discussed why we sometimes find it difficult to keep speed in control. We put it down to enthusiasm about subject, nervousness and forgetfulness. Or maybe a combination of them all. Feedback from practice was good.

Assignment: Purchase weekly train ticket/General phone calls
    Practice asking for ticket, speaking at 180 spm. Make all my morning phone calls at 180 spm (and concentrate on technique).
    Both assignments went well. I found the phone calls, particularly toward lunch time, more difficult to keep under control re speed.

Practice Session — afternoon
Only got 10 minutes to practice, but better than nothing. Discussed results of morning assignment and my afternoon assignment. A little tense about this afternoon's task. Must keep relaxed! Feedback from speech buddy good.

Assignment: Introductions at meeting
I am running two meetings with clients this afternoon and will have to introduce people and give a brief introductory talk. Assignment is to use a high level of technique (desensitising) and not speak over 180 spm.
    Assignments were carried off well. At first I started

to speed up, but managed to pull back and stay at 180 spm. Happy with my level of technique. Felt in full control all the way.

Summary: A demanding speech day — with no problems at all. This is what it's all about!!!

Wednesday, 6 April
Today's Goal: Connection

Practice Session — morning
As part of my overall effort to keep my technique skills sharp, the next area of concentration is to practice the connection between my words. Discussed general technique with speech buddy. Spent around 15 minutes at 100 spm — a slow conversation. Speech buddy having trouble with nerves today. I suggested that he slow down and do some desensitising. We agreed to talk this afternoon to report on each other's progress.

Assignment: No set assignments today — just concentrating on connection and keeping technique sharp.

Practice Session — afternoon
My speech buddy called back and reported that the nervousness had eased a little and that the desensitising assignment (a conversation using obvious technique) had helped.

Summary: It is so easy to let the stutter, or rather fear of it, become so strong that it can really throw you off balance but I must remember — I have the control. It's a question as to how brave I am about exercising it!!!

Let's just quickly go over the main points in this chapter.

1. Practice, practice and then do some more practice — every day. Learn your technique thoroughly.
2. Speak slowly at the beginning. Learn to crawl before you walk.
3. Think out what you are going to say before you speak.
4. Buy a pocket tape-recorder and tape your own speech. Evaluate your assignments with speech buddies.
5. Keep a speech diary.

CHAPTER THREE

DESENSITISING:

GETTING

OVER

THE

EMBARRASSMENT

WHAT IS DESENSITISATION?

It is all very well to have a technique and know how to use it. You may even have mastered the fine arts of controlling speed and thinking before you speak, but without one vital ingredient the whole thing may well come crashing down around your ears. That ingredient is **desensitisation**. I define desensitisation as the ability to use your technique in its most obvious form in any situation without feeling sensitive about it. This may sound a big thing to ask of you, but it is *crucial* if you are going to succeed in overcoming your stutter.

You have your technique and presumably you are skilled at using it. You feel that you have reached your goal of fluency. Sure you stutter, but you now have the knowledge to overcome the stutter. That may be true, but you haven't won out yet! You have to desensitise yourself and this is a real challenge.

We all have pride. It's part of human make-up. Stutterers are no exception. The last thing a stutterer wants to be is different, that is, not to be considered part of the speaking norm. All their stuttering life they have had to deal with being different, then along comes some hope. Yes, you can stop stuttering! *But* you have to use a technique. You will have to speak *differently* from the way you spoke before. You will sound different from everybody else. That degree of difference may alter considerably, depending on the severity of your stutter.

It does not matter how good a technique is. You will not overcome your stutter unless you use it.

You may think everyone in their right mind would use a technique if it could stop them stuttering. But situations occur where pride and fear creep in and all of a sudden using the technique becomes more and more difficult. Let me give you an example.

■ ON THE TRAIL OF FLUENCY

I completed a three week intensive course on fluency shaping. At the completion of the course, I felt I had mastered the technique. My skill in using it was fragile, but I knew I was not going to stutter again and I would be able to speak at 200 syllables per minute. Maybe I would sound a little slurred, but that is a lot better than stuttering. So off I went to face the world knowing that I had cured my stutter. It was only going to be a matter of time before I would be a fluent person in this fluent world.

Everything was fine — until I arrived at work! I realised with a jolt that the commercial world is not really interested in my journey to fluency. The commercial world's primary objective is to make money and I had a job to do and had better get on with it. When I got to work, people were talking at their normal rate of 250–300 spm. The phones were ringing, meetings were being arranged, sales had to be made and on and on it went. I thought that I could gently ease myself into work. Was I wrong! Everyone was talking at me.

'What do you mean you haven't finished it yet?'
'Oh Nick get that phone will you!'
'Come on, Nick, that meeting starts in 10 minutes.'
'Have you got that file I asked for?'
'Nick, grab line 2, Joe can't make 3.00 pm.'
'Nick will you get a move on. The client is downstairs.'
After about a week at work I started to think that

using my technique, that is, speaking at 200 spm and slurring my words, was not going to allow me to survive in my work environment. My technique gives my speech a slurred sound. How can I speak slowly, and sound as though I've been swigging whisky from my hip flask and expect people to take me seriously? What was going to happen when I went into a meeting and had to slow right down and really slur my words to get through a difficult moment without stuttering? I couldn't do it!

Let's look at the situation. You stutter, and as a stutterer you cannot communicate by speech as effectively as someone who does not stutter. Before you put yourself through therapy and learned your technique, you managed in your job, but I bet you had to work hard at it. There were all those moments when you worried about your speech and panicked when you finally struck a bad patch and had to try and push your way through a block. It was not a lot of fun, was it?

Ask yourself these important questions:

- Why do you feel that people will not take what you say seriously when you use the technique?
- Which is more important to you — fluent speech or stuttering?
- Is your job so important that you would jeopardise fluent speech and risk regressing to stuttering for it?

I believe that how you think people will react to your use of a technique and how they actually do react are totally different.

■ OVERCOMING SELF-CONSCIOUSNESS

It is critically important that you desensitise yourself to the use of your technique. You must be able to use it and not feel embarrassed. If you can only avoid stuttering by slowing right down and slurring your words, then that is exactly what you will have to do. It doesn't matter who you are with or what you are doing. Your speech must become your first priority if you are going to overcome your stutter.

You can help desensitise yourself by remembering never to speak without using your technique. You must never stop using your technique even in situations that you are comfortable in. If you do, you will find it very difficult to use the technique in situations that you are *not* comfortable in. If you have not been using your technique continuously, you will find the transition from 'no use' to 'obvious use' difficult. This may mean that your use of your technique is poor and in a formal situation you may find yourself having difficulties. You know what is going to happen. You will stutter! You may then find yourself thinking that your technique does not work. The reality is that your technique works fine. You are just not using it properly.

You have to make a decision once you have completed learning your technique. You have to make it a rule to use it all the time. There can be no exceptions. You can vary the degree by which you slow your speech. If you feel comfortable in a particular situation, you may choose to speak at your maximum speed (220 spm) and you may sound quite normal. In difficult situations, you may need to slow down to say 170–180 spm and increase the level of your technique. Let's look at some practical cases.

When I first started using the technique, I found it difficult to maintain it in work-related situations. I knew that unless 'I bit the bullet' and desensitised myself I would always avoid using the technique because I thought that my speech sounded strange. One day someone in a meeting asked me a question and I blocked. I could not speak. So I stopped altogether. I breathed and then I said to the people in the meeting, 'I have a technique to overcome my stutter and I have not been using it! So I'm going to just take a few moments to get myself together and then I will answer the question'. I expected to be greeted by embarrassment and confusion. Instead people were patient and everybody waited for the 20 seconds or so I needed. Nobody commented on my speech from there on, even though I was using very obvious technique.

Remember. People do not really care what you sound like. It's what you are saying that is important! If that's the case, you may well ask why should you bother making an effort to stop stuttering — it will make you feel better about yourself and if you are speaking slowly and using your technique, you are a lot easier to listen to than someone who is stuttering on every second or third word.

The ability to desensitise yourself to enable you to use your technique is so important that I cannot over emphasise it. It does not matter how much skill or technique you have or therapy you have undergone, you will not be fluent or at the least be able to maintain fluency, unless you have the courage to use your technique.

Here is a scenario with some of the options you might have. You arrive at work on Monday. You have had a relaxing weekend feeling very comfortable. Your speech rate has climbed and you have been able to maintain fluency with little use of technique. On Monday morning at 8.30 am a meeting is called and you have to participate.

You begin with what I call the phantom stutter — you imagine yourself stuttering. You know that if you speak at the speed you used over the weekend, you are going to stutter. You have to decide what to do.

Option 1
You choose to speak quickly and try to sound as normal as possible.

Remember, in this case, if you stutter you are helping your stutter to grow.

Possible outcomes
- You get through the meeting without stuttering. This is highly unlikely and if you got away with it this time, you won't the next time.
- You stutter. It may be a bad block and people will be in no doubt that you have a 'problem' with your speech. They may not invite you to participate next time. In my opinion this is a heavy price to pay.

Option 2
You go into the meeting and speak at 170 spm using obvious technique.

Possible outcome
People think that your natural speech rate is slow. Remember that there are plenty of people whose normal rate is 180–200 spm. You may sound a little different but your audience will forget that quite quickly and start concentrating on what you are saying. After all, this is the reason you are there in the first place. Damage is minimal, if any, in my opinion.

Don't worry what other people will think. Use your technique and slow down. You will not stutter.

HOW TO DESENSITISE YOURSELF

■ VOLUNTARY STUTTERING

Do I really mean this? Yes, I am suggesting that you should stutter deliberately. Think about it. Every time you stuttered in the past, it was because you had no control over your speech. You just talked — and presto, you stuttered. What I am suggesting here is that you practise stuttering on purpose, but that you maintain control. In other words you know exactly what you are doing, how you are doing it, and you know that you can stop stuttering whenever you want to. There are benefits in practising the voluntary stutter.

■ One is you can watch your listener instead of directing all your attention towards getting through a speech block. You can actually feel removed from the situation and see how your listener is responding. This will provide you with valuable information about how people react when you stutter. I am sure you will be surprised. They may not react the way that you think they will.

■ A second benefit is that you will also feel more comfortable. The 'secret' will be out and, quite frankly, who cares? Hopefully you will realise that people accept you even when you stutter, so they are not going to have difficulties accepting you when you use technique, even in its most obvious form.

By using your technique properly and desensitising yourself so that you can use it in all situations, you will be able to communicate freely in any situation. Close your eyes for a minute and think what that really means. Just imagine being at work and being able to concentrate completely on *what* you are saying rather than *how* you are saying it. Imagine how that is going to affect both your performance and your enjoyment! Having a stutter and trying to cope at work is a strain. You use an enormous amount of energy avoiding speech difficulties, worrying and struggling through the day. Imagine that the strain is removed. You can start to focus on your work and not worry so much about your speech.

Desensitise yourself. It's worth the initial embarrassment. You think you sound far worse than you actually do.

Voluntary stuttering is not something that you have to do all the time, just occasionally. If you feel threatened or intimidated by a situation or you feel you cannot use your technique, heed these warning signs. You need to become desensitised, so try a voluntary stutter.

■ SLOWING DOWN

It sounds so simple — and it is. Just slow down. If you feel tense, the chances are you are speaking too quickly. Ignore everybody around you. Controlling your speech is priority number one. Don't worry if your colleagues all speak at 300 spm, and you speak at 180 spm. People will find you far easier to listen to than the 'sprint speaker'.

I personally find it irritating to listen to fast speakers. Listening should be enjoyable, not a physical effort. Usually, when people speak to each other, a kind of fight takes place. If one person speaks more slowly than the other, then one of two things will happen. Either one will speed up, or the other will slow down. You must never enter into that fight. Stay at your own speed. A lot counts on it.

■ DO NOT BE SELF-CONSCIOUS

If you do not desensitise yourself, what can happen is a kind of stuttering catch 22. Let me explain. You approach a situation — let's say it's a meeting and you are aware that you have to speak. You are tense and too self-conscious to use an obvious level of technique. Your tension, combined with your self-consciousness, will probably cause you to start talking too quickly and in the wrong way, that is, without technique. The chances are that you will stutter, and in most cases the reason is your own sensitivity to your stutter. The more often that you find you can talk without stuttering when you're not using your technique, the more self-conscious you become about using it. The only way you can break the cycle is to 'bite the bullet' and use your technique. If you feel as if you are about to stutter, then use more technique to overcome the problem. Remember, that although this may be uncomfortable for you in the beginning, it will prove to be a lot more comfortable for you in the long term.

PRACTISING AT WORK

Another method you can use to become desensitised is to make people aware of your speech technique by doing your practice sessions at work. Here is the sort of thing that I do and what can happen.

I usually arrive at work quite early. This gives me time to do my practice on the phone with my speech buddy (see Chapter 5). I prefer the office for my practice as it gets me used to using my technique in the work environment. I work in an open plan office. My immediate manager sits diagonally opposite me with a partition between us. My director (my manager's boss) sits right behind me with nothing between us. My colleagues sit around me. Essentially everybody can hear everybody else. One morning I was deep in practice, speaking at 150 spm which is very slow compared with normal speech, and certainly very slow compared with the average speed of speech in my work environment. I was slurring away quite loudly as no-one else was in the office.

All of a sudden two of my colleagues appeared, sat down, and proceeded to work. They could hear every word I was saying. I felt very self-conscious. This was a new job, and a job where articulate speech is expected. I continued my practice and I am sure that my speech buddy had no idea that I had people around me. I found practising at work to be of great help in my overall desensitisation. I could just concentrate on what I was saying to my speech buddy and ignore the people around me. I found this gave me a real sense of freedom.

The next time I was on the phone and encountered difficulty I had no trouble in immediately slipping into the use of obvious technique and am now at the stage where I can do it automatically no matter who may be listening. If you find desensitising at work very hard, it means this is the situation in which you probably need desensitising the most. I suggest you try making your practice sessions at work a little louder each time, until it is obvious that people can hear you speak.

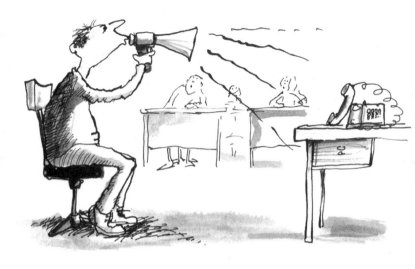

COMMENTS AT WORK

So you have become desensitised! Now that your work colleagues know that you use some kind of speech technique, what are they going to say? The answer is probably — nothing. This is usually not a big deal to anybody but you. Today, people are very tolerant of other people's habits and attitudes. We all realise that the 'perfect person' is a myth.

How people respond to you depends on who you work with and what your general situation is. I can only speak for myself. I have found that if people do say anything it is usually out of interest. They may ask if I stutter and how long I have done so. They may make comments about someone they know who stutters and so on. Then it is usually forgotten. All that panic I felt, all that fear I carried around — for what? For nothing. Learning to become desensitised is one of the most important things you can do, whether you have had treatment or not.

Looking at the 'why' of stuttering

When anyone receives information, they only comprehend what fits within their boundaries of understanding. All other information will pass uncomprehended. We can explain this phenomenon by using an analogy. You may be familiar with the drawing of a woman's silhouette in which some people see a young woman, others see an old woman. This difference can be attributed to the individual's perception. But what has this to do with stuttering and speech?

It's all to do with how we perceive a particular situation and what our experience or history has been when we've been confronted with that, or a similar situation before. If from past experience you know that in a particular situation you will stutter, all information that supports stuttering in this situation is allowed through to your consciousness. All information that supports fluent speech in this situation is blocked out. I am no expert on psychology but I can remember with painful clarity being in situations in which, before I have been called upon to speak, I have known with absolute certainty that I was going to stutter. And guess what happened? I stuttered!

My perception was controlling the situation. It was supporting my belief that all the information available to me was telling me that I was going to stutter. It did not allow the information that would support fluency in that situation to surface.

Now you know as well as I do that you are not going to stop stuttering overnight. However, I can assure you that changing your idea of what is achievable or what you feel is acceptable to others is going to make a tremendous difference to the progress that you make towards fluency and how you feel about yourself generally. But how can you do this? Throughout this guide I mention the importance of replacing negative experiences with positive ones and the importance of desensitising yourself to achieve this.

It would be unrealistic to suggest that you will gain complete confidence quickly. It is going to take a lot of time and a lot of work. One thing you can do which will help speed this process is to remove the fear associated with particular situations and replace it with feelings of confidence. This will help promote fluency. You must teach yourself to believe that you have control over your speech and shut out the negative voices that tell you you will stutter in a particular situation.

You have all the skills needed to speak fluently. Practise using these until they become second nature.

As you approach a situation that you find stressful — try and take a few moments to analyse why you are feeling so uptight. Perhaps you are considering all the negative aspects of the situation rather than the positive.

Negative aspects such as your history — similar situations to the one you are about to enter where you have stuttered — come flooding back into your memory. You walk into the room, your confidence escapes you, you suddenly feel that you have lost control, the work that you did to learn your technique goes out the window and you stutter. The battle was lost before you even opened your mouth, wasn't it? Your mental approach to the situation is vitally important.

Instead of walking into the situation with sweaty palms and knocking knees try thinking about it from another perspective. Rather than getting really nervous about the situation, realise that the choice to speak fluently or stutter is yours to make. You have control over your speech. No-one else has!

The only questions in your mind should be what level of technique you should use and at what speed you should speak to guarantee that you do not stutter. If you feel that you cannot use high level technique or slow right down, then you need to practise becoming desensitised. Do not fear situations. Know that you can get through any situation that you want to. It's up to you.

■ THE STUTTERING LOOP

I believe that a kind of mental 'loop' occurs before you actually stutter. It is during this loop that you convince yourself that you are going to stutter on a particular word. You have to realise that the grey matter in your head is like a computer. It is not only powerful but is also very obliging — and will do exactly what you tell it to.

If you are talking with someone and you are speaking fluently and using your technique, something like this can occur. You can go from fluency to a stutter in the matter of a millisecond. I have based my explanation of the stuttering loop on what happens to me. But I have spoken with a lot of stutterers and there seems to be general agreement that they know they are going to stutter a split second before they do. This does not happen all the time, but it does happen some of the time.

The beginning of the 'loop' is triggered by speed. As soon as you allow your fluency and comfort level to distract you from concentrating on your technique, you

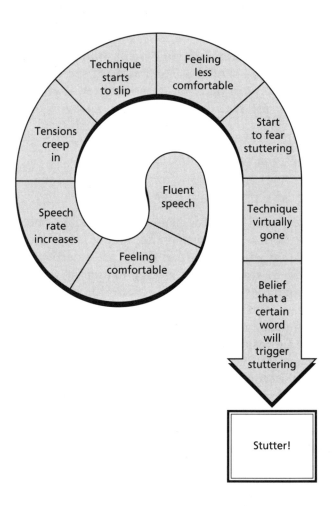

risk going into the 'loop', and it can happen so fast that it's virtually impossible to stop. The moral of the story is: do not start the process. Keep your mind on your technique and your speed *at all times*. I would suggest that as soon as you feel comfortable, that is when you should be on the alert.

TACKLING DIFFICULT SITUATIONS

It is important that you try to engage in speaking situations that you would normally find difficult or threatening. Do not push yourself so hard that you will end up with a negative experience, but at the same time, try to avoid relaxing in a comfort zone.

When you look at a difficult speaking situation, you may initially feel that it is too great a step for you to take at this time. Be careful not to let your 'fear' (which is falsely based on previous experience, not on 'technique-based' experience) wrongly influence you.

For instance, let's say that you work for a company that continually runs a program of presentations for the benefit of its clients. It engages a professional speaker to give the presentation and it is the responsibility of the members of staff to introduce the speaker and present a short sales pitch about the organisation. We will assume that performing introductions is purely a voluntary role and there is no pressure on the staff to volunteer. You believe that this would be an excellent 'speech assignment' for yourself but you are nervous about participating because you feel that you will stutter. What do you do?

Your feeling of nervousness is likely to be due to your belief that others will not accept your use of high level

35

technique in this situation. Because you believe this, your degree of control is reduced and you therefore feel that you are likely to stutter. The loss of control, or rather the belief that you have lost control, starts the 'old' thought processes and sets you up for stuttering.

Let's analyse the situation. Your colleagues and management, a guest speaker and clients are all present. The presentations may well be held in a formal type of environment such as a convention room or possibly a lecture room. This is a difficult situation because you quite naturally feel pressured by the fact that your speech may fail you in front of people who are very important to your career.

You need to reduce the 'speech nervousness' associated with this occasion. You can achieve this by taking two steps.

- The first is to prepare for the presentation (see Chapter 7).
- The second is to start using a high level of technique at work in front of those colleagues who are likely to be attending the presentation. This will desensitise you to using obvious technique so you will not feel so self-conscious using this level of technique during the presentation.

Remember that your colleagues will have heard you practising your technique. They know what you sound like. If they are comfortable at the thought of your using a high level of technique, and of being involved in the presentation, then you should be also.

The reason you need to use high level technique on this occasion is because this is a difficult speech task. You will have to build up to it slowly. You may need to do several less threatening tasks before you can tackle this sort of speaking situation with a lower level of technique. You have shown that you can speak fluently in this situation, albeit with heavy technique, but at least you were speaking fluently. Everyone could understand you perfectly. This is a significant improvement on pre-technique days.

If you are still concerned about using high level technique during the presentation then bring the matter up at the next meeting. Make everybody aware of what you see as the problem. I would suggest that you do not describe the problem as *your* problem, but rather that you may need to use an obvious level of technique should you encounter difficulties and ask whether this causes your colleagues any concern.

A good idea at this point may be to rehearse the presentation using an obvious level of technique in front of your colleagues. Then ask whether they agree to your doing the presentation.

I am confident that your colleagues will agree that you should do the presentation. If they decide that you should not, do not be disheartened. Consider what you have achieved. In discussing the situation with your colleagues and using an obvious level of technique during the rehearsal presentation, you have taken a major step in desensitising yourself. These are significant achievements. Well done!

It is very important to realise what you can and cannot manage. It is better to make an approach to a task using an obvious level of technique than to go ahead hoping you can bluff your way through and end up stuttering. That will be a far greater setback than being told you cannot give a presentation because you intend using a speech technique.

If your colleagues say no to you on this occasion, accept their judgement. Pat yourself on the back for having desensitised yourself further and for showing that you have control over your speech, not your speech over you. Suggest to your colleagues that you try again later. Do not forget to tell your speech buddies about your great efforts when you next call them.

If your colleagues agree to your giving the presentation, you must not under any circumstances reduce your level of technique.

I suggest that the day before the presentation and certainly on the day itself, you should speak at the level of technique you intend to use for the presentation. This may or may not be practical for you. It is a good idea, however, because it will make you feel more comfortable using it and will increase your chances of being able to use the technique at this level throughout the whole of the presentation. Now read 'The presentation' in Chapter 7.

■ REPLACING NEGATIVE FEELINGS WITH POSITIVE FEELINGS

> 'Oh, I woke up this mornin'
> went to say hello to you . . .
> Oh I woke up this mornin'
> went to say I love you.
> Opened up my mouth to find
> I had those old stuttering blues'

I may not be a great blues song writer, but you will understand what I'm saying. Having a stutter can really get you down. It's not your fault you stutter, is it? So you have a right to be angry about it, right? **WRONG!**

Open your eyes, take a deep breath, thank God you're alive and let's talk. You stutter. This is probably genetic. I know that stuttering can be a painful affliction, but at least you can see and walk and feel and think. So forget about anger. It is a totally negative emotion. Consider your situation and then do something positive about it.

The thoughts you carry around in your head are possibly part of your problem. Why do you perceive speaking situations the way you do? What sort of thoughts go buzzing around in your head before you stutter? You have to work on replacing those negative 'fear' feelings with positive reinforcing ones. This may take some soul-searching and some time, but you will probably gain some really interesting insights, not just into your stutter, but into yourself.

Let's revise the key points of this chapter.

1. Examine your options regarding your speech. Do not let any misconceptions you may have about what you sound like stop you from using your technique.

2. Try to desensitise yourself. I am sure it won't be as painful as you thought it might be.

The important methods you can use to become desensitised are:

- voluntary stuttering
- slowing down your speech rate
- practising at work.

Most importantly, don't give a thought to how other people might perceive the way you sound. You think you sound far worse than you actually do.

STARVING

THE

STUTTER

When you think about it, stuttering is a very strange thing! In all other respects stutterers are perfectly 'normal'. Sometimes they do not stutter. Some stutterers are perfectly fluent when they are angry or when they have had a few drinks. The stutter seems to come and go, depending on the situation or perhaps on the stutterer's perception of the situation.

I mentioned in Chapter 3 how important desensitising yourself is to the success of whatever technique you employ to maintain your fluency. You should be able to adjust the level of technique according to how you are feeling and how likely you are to stutter. Just as important as the ability to use your technique in its most obvious form is the ability to stop thinking like a stutterer.

FOUR TABOOS

I'm not suggesting here that you do not think about your stutter — quite the contrary. You must always be aware of your stutter and your technique. However, there are certain little tricks that you and I as stutterers are very good at using, which unfortunately act as food for the stutter and help it grow.

What I want you to concentrate on at the moment are certain negative tactics that you should learn to recognise and overcome if you find yourself using them.

They are:

- **word avoidance**
- **situation avoidance**
- **spontaneous fluency**
- **use of filler words.**

Let's cover these in more detail.

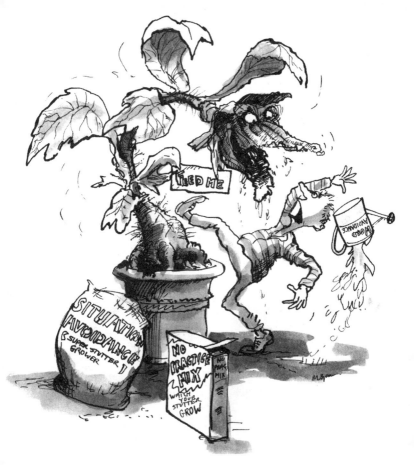

■ WORD AVOIDANCE

Remember when you stuttered every time you opened your mouth? Then you developed little tricks to get around the stutter, so that you could at least retain some of your dignity and get a few words out. You have probably refined that system to an art form.

One of the most effective methods that I used, and I know a lot of other stutterers have as well, is **word**

43

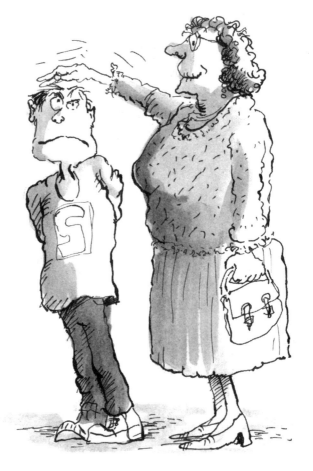

avoidance. The trick here is to replace a word you cannot say with a 'user friendly' word, that is, one you *can* say. I used to do it all the time. When I was 17, I couldn't say the word 'seventeen'. It was amazing how many people would ask me how old I was! So I kept saying that I would be 18 in so many months. Some of the older women thought that was cute, most people thought I was rather strange, but *I* thought it certainly beat stuttering.

As time goes by, we stutterers develop an enormous vocabulary of user friendly words and become masters at slipping them in, just in the nick of time. Sometimes they don't exactly fit into the sentence, but using them is a lot better than stuttering. Now I know this is like saying goodbye to an old friend, but we have to stop using this vocabulary of words that we have grown to love and cherish. They are not helping us!

Imagine that your stutter is a huge noxious weed. Every time you practise word avoidance, you throw a bucket of fertiliser on it. Every time you successfully replace a bad experience with a good one, that is, you are fluent, you chop a bit off the weed.

You use word avoidance because when you are speaking, that little panic machine in your mind goes racing ahead and flags all the trouble words. For example, it can happen when you get asked a question.

Let's say you are 27 years old and you work at Sammy Seal's Supermarket. Now let's imagine that you have trouble with 's' words. (It might be wise to get a job somewhere else!) People will often ask you how old you are and where you work. So you have probably developed a little system to get around using the 's' words. When asked how old you are, you probably say, 'I'm nearly 30', or 'not quite 30'. But what do you say when asked where you work? You can handle this in two ways. If the person is not likely to know Sammy Seal's Supermarket, you can probably get away with saying something like 'in a big grocery store'. If they *are* likely to know Sammy Seal's, you will probably answer, 'that big grocery store in town' and it's up to the listener to provide the name. And you get angry with them, don't you when they cannot work it out and keep asking you for the name?

After this little dialogue has come to some sort of an end, you thank God you managed to avoid that potential stutter. But all you have done is avoided saying words that will come up again and again. You have reinforced your chances of stuttering on those words next time.

You often think that you are a social idiot because of your word avoidance. Your listener may be confused about you — it depends on how well you managed the context. So at seventeen when I was asked my age and I answered, 'I'll be eighteen in eleven months', it probably sounded a bit strange. This type of word avoidance makes you all the more anxious. So what should you do?

First, **no more word avoidance**. If you feel that you are going to stutter on a word, it is *not* the word that's the problem — it is you. You are not using your technique properly. As a technique, I use fluency shaping, which basically means I slow down, concentrate on breathing, phrasing and linking my words together. If during a conversation I find I am getting tense, particularly about 's' sounds, which were always my weakness, I treat this as a warning sign that something is wrong with my use of the technique. When I come upon a word that I feel I will stutter on, I stop, breathe and start off again very slowly and then build up to my usual speed.

Second, **do not worry about the listener**. Let listeners make up their own mind about you and your speech. It is of no importance whether they think you sound strange or not. Consider how they would be coping if they stuttered. Having a stutter is not a crime. It is not something that has been inflicted on you for some heinous act. You are coping with your stutter as best you can. The listener will cope too. If you feel that you are going to stutter on a word, then do whatever is necessary for you to say the word according to your technique. You may decide to stop and start again. You may decide to stutter on purpose. But under no circumstance should you avoid using the problem word. If you do, you will be adding to the problem, not taking away from it.

In some situations, you fear answering certain questions because the answers will contain your 'trouble' words as a component (such as our Sammy Seal's example). In these circumstances, I suggest that you prepare your answers and become familiar with answering these questions using your technique. Practising your answers increases your level of desensitisation. Remember, under no circumstances use word avoidance.

If you find you still do this, write the problem word in your speech diary (see Chapter 2) and refer to it when you next talk to your speech buddies (see Chapter 5). Plan to use that word in situations you have more control over. This will increase the good experience associated with it, rather than the bad.

Practising word avoidance can lead you along strange paths. I did an accountancy degree at university. I was very relieved when I finished it, not because I found it intellectually difficult, but because it presented problems for my speech. You will all recognise the words 'asset', 'liability', 'debit' and 'credit' as the cornerstones of the accounting language. And these were the very words that I found most difficult to say. So I made up substitutes!

One day I was put in the miserable position of having to explain a problem to the class, and what did I have to talk about? Assets, liabilities, debits and credits. So I used my substitutes and an astonished class heard me explain double entry bookkeeping in terms of 'good things on the left and bad things on the right'. Even now, I remember the expression of complete disbelief on the lecturer's face and the amused looks I got from my fellow students. I came away from that class contemplating my life as an unemployed accountant!

■ SITUATION AVOIDANCE

Do you recognise this scenario? You are at work and your particular group, department or team is to hold a seminar. Some people from your group will be required to give presentations. Let us assume that can usually cope, that is to say, sometimes you may stutter, but most of the time you will get by. You have achieved this by using word avoidance and situation avoidance. You don't want to expose yourself as a stutterer in front of everybody. As long as you can avoid situations that may lead to a public discovery you think you will be all right.

Let's talk a little on situation avoidance in a career. My professional career over the last ten years or so has been in sales. To be successful in sales requires many things, one of which is opportunity. In order to make opportunities in your life you have to be visible. By visible, I mean people in your organisation and people in your market who are your future customers, have to know you and what you do. Being visible often requires being at the lectern talking to a group. Are stutterers going to put themselves in this position? No. They are most likely going to avoid the situation.

Let's look at this a bit more closely. Let's assume you are a stutterer and you are in sales. 'Why sales?' you ask. 'Why not something that does not require as much fluent speech?' I think it would be reasonable to assume you are in sales because you enjoy it, are proficient at it and can make a living from it. We will assume that you are doing well at your sales career because you are reasonably fluent.

Let's say that hardly anyone in the company other than those who work with you knows that you stutter. So getting up and talking to the company and customers would mean that your secret would be out.

What goes through your mind when people are asked to volunteer to give the presentation? Not many people like public speaking, but it is the people who become visible in their company and to their clients who seem to get the rewards. You probably dread being asked to do a presentation. If people are being asked to volunteer, you will probably try to hide and wait for someone else to volunteer. Quite possibly you justify your action by thinking 'it's a waste of time. I'm better off concentrating on other aspects of the job'.

This is not true. It is not a waste of time! It will be of benefit to your career to volunteer for the presentation. In fact, avoiding doing presentations may well stop you from reaching your goals in the company, and it will also make you feel mentally separated from those in the company who *do* give presentations.

As well as this, avoiding the situation can lead you to think that you do not deserve your job because you feel you cannot provide the full service that the others can.

I feel confident that those company representatives who do not promote themselves and do not become visible within the company may not succeed as well as those who do. I believe that you can give the presentation. In fact I also believe that you may possibly give a better presentation than the others, if only because you will have to work considerably harder at the preparation (see Chapter 7, 'The presentation').

I've been talking about situation avoidance when you are pursuing a career. But what of the ordinary situations that arise when you are young and unsure of yourself?

I remember my early experiences with girls, when I used to feel that being found out as a stutterer would be the end of my world! To pretend that I spoke like everybody else, I avoided using words I knew I had trouble with and I tried not to get into situations that would cause me to lose control of my speech. I remember doing a lot of discreet swallowing of air to try and avoid stuttering in front of a girlfriend.

Taking a girlfriend to the movies was one of my situation avoidance ploys. Movies solved a lot of my problems. It was a place where my girlfriend and I could sit and silently enjoy the film. I could relax. I did not have to talk! What blissful relief from trying to hide the fact that I stuttered. Did I ever see a lot of movies in those days — more I think than the critics did!

Avoiding situations because of fear is not going to help your career or your stutter. Do not push yourself into situations that overcommit you, but at the same time, do not avoid situations because of a wrongly based fear.

■ SPONTANEOUS FLUENCY

Quite possibly you were taught the technique that you now use in a controlled clinic environment over a period of weeks and feel you have become fully fluent. You may have been saturated with fluency enhancing techniques and support. Unfortunately, a strange phenomenon can occur as a result of this kind of intensive treatment. The best way to describe spontaneous fluency is as a fluency hangover. You can literally walk out of the clinic at the conclusion of the treatment and because you and the clinicians have been paying so much attention to your speech, you experience a high degree of natural fluency. I describe this as 'natural' because it can come without any work. You just open your mouth and you speak fluently.

It would give me great joy to be able to report that this phenomenon lasts a long time, but unfortunately it doesn't. Not only does it desert you but, if you rely on it, it can rob you of the first few weeks when it is crucial that you consolidate your technique.

This is what happens when you speak with this spontaneous fluency. You start speaking and very quickly speed up until you are speaking at your natural rate, or even faster. In my case this would be at around 270 spm, in other words, very fast. As the stutter starts to recur you arrive at what I call speech dead ends. One minute you will be speaking fluently at 270 spm and the next you will try to say a word and nothing comes out. All you can really do is to start again and use your technique to get over the block.

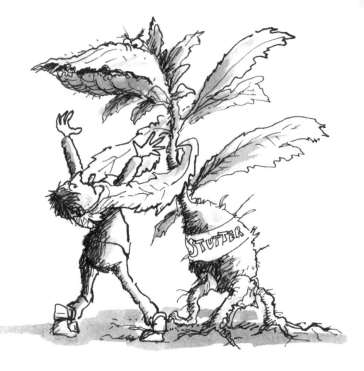

This is probably the last thing you will do because you will be in a state of shock, realising that this newly found fluency has deserted you as suddenly as it found you.

I believe this spontaneous fluency has been responsible for many post-treatment regressions. When I did my first intensive treatment session at the age of 18, I came out after two weeks of live-in therapy, totally fluent. I was on top of the world. At that time very little was done to help stutterers maintain their fluency. I was so overjoyed at being able to speak without stuttering that I just talked and talked and talked. Slowly but surely my stutter woke from its nap and started to wrap its hand around my throat. It did not take long before I was back where I started. Actually I was worse off than when I started since

I now believed I would never overcome my stutter. I had devoted two full weeks of my life to 12-hour days of therapy and where had it got me? If I had had the knowledge to *maintain* my new fluency, it would have significantly improved my quality of life.

If you are to maintain your fluency, it is absolutely critical that you use your technique after you finish treatment. Recognise this initial period of fluency without effort for what it is — 'fools gold' fluency.

■ FILLER SOUNDS

One other thing everyone has to beware of is using filler words. Words such as 'well' are usually unnecessary in the context of what you are saying. Often they are used as a means to start speaking when you are feeling tense. That in itself is not a real problem. It only becomes a problem when you start to use 'well' as a support mechanism. Filler sounds such as 'er', 'ah' and 'um' should be avoided. They can trigger stuttering. Unfortunately nearly everybody uses filler sounds, often unconsciously.

I believe the best way to eliminate the use of filler sounds is to speak more slowly, and to think before you speak. Get that imaginary screen working for you.

Think back to the days when you were a chronic stutterer and could not get out the word you wanted. If you could just magically listen to a tape-recording of your speech from those days, what you would probably hear just prior to stuttering is a lot of filler words, particularly 'ums' and 'ers'. I believe a reason for this is that, prior to stuttering, you have flagged the word that you are going to stutter on and you use the filler sounds (the 'ums' and 'ers') as a kind of running jump to the word. Or perhaps you have reached a block and the only sound you can get out is 'um' or 'er'. It is amazing how quickly this can become a habit and reinforce stuttering.

Let's look at a practical example. I have trouble with the word *cinema*. So what does a friend ask me?

'Hi Nick, where are you going tonight?'

'I'm going to the . . . um . . . er . . . um . . . cin . . . um . . . cinema.'

I have got the word out, but I used the filler sounds as my springboard. They also provided me with some sounds to feed to my listener, because I felt that a pause whilst I was desperately trying to push the sound out would be unacceptable.

The object of this guide is to help you maintain fluency. Don't use anything in your speech that disrupts fluency. Filler sounds do not communicate anything. Try to avoid using them. Regard them as your enemies.

To avoid using filler sounds:

- slow down
- think of what you are going to say before you speak. (Use your personal screen.)

OVERCOMPENSATING AT WORK

> 'Hey . . . I stutter . . . I have to work harder
> than anybody else . . . I have to hold this job
> down somehow!'
>
> An overworked, anonymous stutterer

I started my career as an accountant. All of my aptitude tests showed I had a high level of numeracy skill and this led to my taking up accountancy. The problem for me was not in calculating figures, but in saying them, particularly over the phone. I remember I would often prefer to drive somewhere to meet clients so that I could relay information in person rather than use the phone. This was not exactly good time management! The other accountants around me all sounded so knowledgeable and professional. I had all the knowledge, but when it came to giving my manager financial information, I didn't *sound* really knowledgeable.

I spent some time as an accountant for a prestigious art gallery in London, a job I really loved. The gallery was a really 'flexible' place; it had to be, dealing with artists all day, so I thought they would be tolerant towards my stutter — and they were. The trustees of the gallery, most of whom were lord and earls, were very influential and well-known figures in England. Every three months the directors and the accountant of the gallery had to present the financial affairs to the Board of Trustees.

There I was sitting in the beautiful regal boardroom surrounded by the who's who of England being asked to interpret the balance sheet. As I stuttered along, two things were occupying my mind. Firstly, the desire to give up accountancy and take a job where I didn't have to talk. Secondly, how to get out of the room as quickly as possible. But I struggled through. Afterwards I felt that I had lowered the dignity of the gallery. To make up for this, I worked and worked to try and regain the respect of the board. What complete nonsense! It was stupid to feel that I had let anybody down. Why should I feel ashamed?

Do you overwork to compensate for your stutter? If it is a Sunday and you are at the office processing the work of two people because you feel that speech-wise you are only half a person, my advice is to stop. Think seriously about your situation. First of all, you have a job. Either you have been with the company for some time and have risen to this position or you have recently applied for the position and have been appointed. You were chosen over everybody else. The company has recognised your talents and abilities. Sure, you may stutter when you are not using your technique properly, but I am sure that is well known in the company. Relax. You do not have to prove anything to anybody.

If you honestly believe that, because you stutter, you have to put in a superhuman effort to keep your job, then you should be reassessing your job. You will not live a balanced life if you spend all your time at work. Family relationships and your health may suffer and these are at least as important as work.

If you feel that you are overcompensating at work, reread the chapter on desensitising yourself. Learn to speak with your technique. Stop thinking you are inadequate and enjoy a more balanced approach to your work. If you manage to achieve this, you will quite possibly find you are doing your job even better than before.

Remember the following rules.

- Do not use word avoidance
- Do not use situation avoidance
- Stop worrying about the listener
- Be on the look out for spontaneous fluency
- Forget the 'ums' and 'ers'
- Stop feeling that you have to do the work of two people because you stutter.

No one likes rules, but having rules can often be a help in certain situations. Following these ones can help improve your speech.

CHAPTER FIVE

YOU AND YOUR SPEECH BUDDIES

You may have felt throughout your life as a stutterer that you have been alone — that nobody understands exactly what you are going through to ease the pain of your situation. For the sake of your fluency this has to change. There is absolutely no reason in the world why you have to be alone. You are about to undertake an enormous challenge and change your natural way of speaking.

Most stutterers know other stutterers. If you do not, get in touch with whatever treatment centres or speech groups you can find and make contact with some stutterers. They will become your speech buddies.

Try and get together with two other stutterers. Make sure that they are totally familiar with your technique and that they share your dedication and commitment to fluent speaking.

Do not think you can overcome stuttering on your own. You will find that there are many occasions when you need either support or the evaluation of others to keep you going, and going in the right direction. Attaining fluency is going to take everything you have got. It is absolutely imperative that you have people around who can support you.

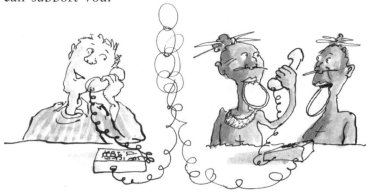

WHAT YOU NEED FROM SPEECH BUDDIES

- *Evaluation.* You will need other people who fully understand your technique to evaluate and criticise your use of it.

  An informed outsider's opinion can sometimes put you back on course, when you did not even realise you had strayed.

- *A shoulder to cry on.* You need this when things go wrong — and they will! Even normal fluent speakers have times in their speaking day when fluency deserts them. There will inevitably be situations that cause you high anxiety. These will affect your use of the technique and consequently your level of fluency. When this happens you need a shoulder to cry on and, more importantly, someone to help you analyse why things went wrong.

- *Praise.* When you succeed in a difficult situation — and if you follow your technique you should have plenty of successes — then celebrate! Laugh about it. You have met the challenge and won out in a potentially bad situation. You need to share these moments with your speech buddies and they need to share theirs with you.

- *Daily practice.* You will need people to practise your technique with. I believe that you will get better results from practising your speech with a speech buddy than with someone who has never stuttered. You need someone who can be brutally honest with you, someone who knows all the little tricks you are likely to use and also someone who can really understand the achievement when you get the results you were aiming for.

How my speech buddy group formed

I attended a three-week full-time course of treatment at a clinic in Australia. There were four of us booked in for treatment. We all started on a Monday. By the following Wednesday one had dropped out leaving the three of us to carry on. During the ensuing two and a half weeks, a special bond developed between us. As we were all striving together to attain fluency we became good friends and these friendships have lasted to this day.

After we finished the treatment, we agreed that we would form a support group. We arranged to call each other every day to practise our technique and we agreed to discuss problems and successes when these occurred. We religiously maintained contact and to this day this support is as important to the three of us as the learning of the technique itself was.

Over the following years, my circle of speech buddies has enlarged considerably. Although I still maintain contact with my two original buddies, I now speak regularly to five speech buddies. No matter how busy we may be, we always find time for each other. Sometimes a couple of minutes can make a world of difference to our speech for that day.

One of my speech buddies rang me the other day just before she had to make a presentation at work. We spent about ten minutes going over part of the text. She was speaking far too quickly, probably because she was nervous. I managed to get her to focus on her technique and to concentrate on slowing her speech rate down. I also suggested that during her talk she visualise the room full of speech buddies, with me at the front monitoring her speed. Her presentation was such a success that some of the people present congratulated her on the way she spoke.

Calling me just prior to giving the presentation enabled my friend to get everything back on track. This quite possibly turned a potentially negative situation into a positive one.

Use your speech buddies. It is a two-way street. Be there for them and they will be there for you.

THE IMPORTANCE OF PRACTICE

■ DAILY PRACTICE

You must practise your technique *every day*. The skills that you have acquired are extremely fragile after treatment and daily practice is needed to strengthen them. You have been stuttering for a long time, so developing new skills is going to be quite a battle. I practise on the telephone with my speech buddies for at least 30 minutes every day. I very rarely miss a practice session because I know that if I do, I start to fall into bad habits. A stutter is a very insidious thing. It is often quite happy to lie around and wait for you to slip up. If you do not commit yourself to a regime of daily practice you will start to make mistakes and go back to your old way of speaking — which is stuttering.

HOW TO PRACTISE

Every morning before you start your day, set aside 30 minutes to go through your speech exercises. If possible you should do these exercises with someone who under-stands your technique, preferably a speech buddy.

As I have said earlier, I use the fluency shaping technique. It is based on speed of speech, breathing and pausing, the linking of words together and the use of soft onsets to the sounds when you start to speak. So in order to keep my technique skills sharp, I do the following practice exercises, but your practice may differ depending on what your technique requires.

- Firstly, I concentrate on my breathing, being aware of my inhaling and exhaling. As I focus on my breathing I consider my speech, imagining that I am speaking as I exhale the air from my lungs. This exercise helps me concentrate on my breathing.

- Secondly, I start speaking very slowly, accentuating the syllables and concentrating on connecting each word so that they are all linked. I remember to start my speaking on the exhaling breath, to phrase my words and to pause.

- Thirdly, I gradually speed up my speech, spending at least five minutes at each speed. I finally arrive at the desired speed for my speech.

These are the speeds I use during my practice session.

100 syllables per minute
This is a very slow speed. At this rate I sound like a 45 record played at 33⅓ rpm. My speech is very slurred. This is a good exercise for concentrating on the connection between words and on the technique skills generally.

150 syllables per minute
This is still slow. I pay special attention to phrasing and pausing.

180–200 syllables per minute
This may be the speed that I choose to speak at for the day. At 180 spm, speech should sound quite normal except

for a slight amount of slurring. Once I am speaking at 180–200 spm I select somebody that I feel comfortable with, such as a neighbour or colleague, who does not know that I am practising my technique. This will make the conversation more realistic. I telephone them and concentrate on my technique as I speak.

This final exercise is very important, as its purpose is to 'set' my speech pattern for the day. If I do not do this I may find that even after doing my practice, I run the risk of entering my first speaking situation of the day without adequate technique. If I have had a 'controlled' conversation to begin with, it gives me an 'anchor' for the day.

I try to set aside a practice period for the afternoon as well as the morning. I said earlier that following this guide would test your patience and determination, but controlling a stutter is not easy. And you are going to have to practise your speech technique at least once a day from this day on. You will constantly have to monitor your speech and every time you open your mouth you must use your technique. It's hard, but it gets easier as it becomes more automatic. I cannot put enough stress on this need for total commitment.

WHAT IF THE PRACTICE DOES NOT WORK?

If you are still stuttering, then you are not using your technique! I know of stutterers who practise and practise but still have problems. Other stutterers may use their technique brilliantly in certain situations but when they get to work, they find they are stuttering again. They shrug their shoulders and say 'well, the technique only works some of the time, and I've always had trouble at work!'.

Let's look at this situation rationally. The problem is either that you do not know how to use your technique, which is unlikely if you are carrying out your practice or, for some reason, you are not using your technique. If after a lot of practice you are still experiencing difficulties, either you have not learned your technique correctly and are reinforcing your incorrect use of it, or you have not become desensitised in those situations that you are still finding difficult.

It is unlikely that you have learned your technique incorrectly, particularly if you were trained by professionals. It is far more likely that you are not allowing yourself to use your technique in certain situations. This could be attributable to lack of desensitisation. If you find that in some situations you speak perfectly fluently and in others you stutter, it is reasonable to assume that you have a desensitisation problem. You need to review your use of technique and your level of desensitisation in those 'trouble' situations. Let's use these 'hot spots' to design a practice program.

■ A HIERARCHY OF ASSIGNMENTS

The dictionary definition of a 'hierarchy' is an organisation with grades ranked one above another. I am going to list at least ten speaking situations as a hierarchy. Number 10, the easiest, is at the bottom of the hierarchy, and the hardest, which is listed as number 1, is at the top. It is important that you give some real thought to these speech situations because this is going to be the blueprint of your assignment program.

You are going to work through each speaking

situation, moving on to the next only when you are satisfied that you have control over the earlier situation.

Here is an example of a hierarchy of speaking situations.
1. Giving a presentation at work
2. Participating in a meeting at work
3. Making a telephone call at work
4. Having a conversation at work
5. Making introductions at work
6. Making social introductions
7. Making a telephone call to a stranger
8. Talking to a friend on the telephone
9. Having a conversation with a friend
10. Ordering lunch in a public place.

This grading of situations gives you an idea of how to set up a hierarchy. When you have worked out a 10 step hierarchy that suits the sorts of situations you encounter, your next step is to set yourself an assignment, starting with the easiest.

ASSIGNMENTS

Step 10 in our hierarchy example is ordering lunch in a public place. This is a reasonably easy situation to cope with, but can on occasions cause some difficulty. The plan is to prepare for this situation so that you are in control of your speech. In order to move to the next step, you have to successfully tackle step 10 according to whatever criteria you decide on. You may, for example, decide that you will repeat step 10 until you are confident that you have full control of your speech or until you are satisfied that your skills are being used correctly and fully. This may mean that you order what you actually *want* for lunch instead of what you find easy to say!

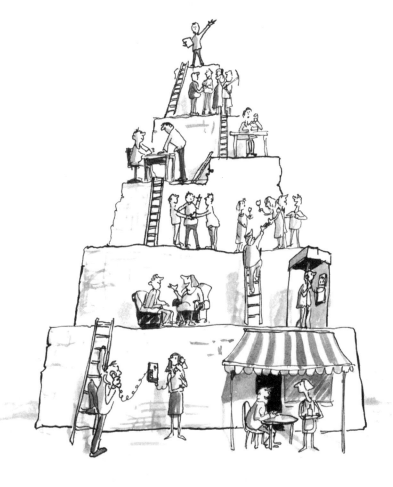

THE ASSIGNMENT SHEET

It is important to record the assignment. The assignment sheet given suits my particular needs. You should draft something that suits your particular needs. The assignment sheet below is based on the fluency shaping technique and lists the components relevant to my technique. In the skills box, list the components relevant to *your* technique.

Assignment Sheet
Date:

Hierarchy Grade
State what step on the hierarchy you attempted.

Situation
Describe the situation you practised in.

Skills

1. Speed (spm) Write down how many syllables per minute you were speaking. If you are unsure of your speed ask your speech buddies what they think the speed was, after they have listened to the recording. (See page 14 'Recording your speech.')

2. Breathing Were you breathing smoothly and consistently? Did you start each phrase as you exhaled? Did you let the sound out as you began speaking?

3. Phrasing Were you phrasing your words properly? As a guide to monitoring your speed, note how many syllables you are speaking in a phrase.

4. Pausing Were you pausing? How often were you pausing and for how long?

5. Connecting Were you connecting all the words in your sentences or were the words separate? Your words should be linked together and come out smoothly.

6. Thinking Did you think before you spoke? Did you visualise the words before you began to say them?

Comments

■ What was good? State what, in regard to your speech, you think was the part of the assignment you did best.

■ What was bad? Note areas in which you felt your speech could be improved.

EXAMPLES OF ASSIGNMENTS

Here are some examples of the assignments that I have put myself through.

'S' word assignment

As I have mentioned earlier, I had trouble with 's' sounding words. I thought that carrying out assignments based on 's' words would show up any problems that might be occurring with regard to my technique.

I selected a retail area (in this case, a mall in the centre of Sydney) and went from shop to shop. I intended to cover enough shops to get a full 30 minutes of recorded speech. This is how I proceeded.

I introduced myself and explained that my grand-mother was in the habit of putting deposits on goods that she did not want and then forgetting where she had paid the deposit. This, of course, left her grandson with the task of trying to retrace her steps in order to discover the shop that held her deposit and hopefully get it back.

The name of 'my grandmother' was Sharon Sheridan, which for me was a great test of 's' sounds. The deposit was always 'seventy dollars'.

Keep making your assignments harder so they will test you and also show up any weaknesses that may be creeping in. Be creative with your assignments. It makes them more fun. Do not forget to put your tape-recorder on, so that you can evaluate your performance afterwards. Good luck!

Shopping assignment

Here is a suggested assignment in case you cannot think of any yourself. My suggestion is based on speech sounds that you might find difficult. I would recommend that you design your own, based on your own areas of difficulty, but if you prefer, you can try the one suggested.

Pick two or three sounds or words you find difficult to say. These may be 'f', 'th', 'm' or 's' for example.

Here's the scenario. You are shopping for furniture. Explain to the sales assistant that you have a federation style home, or a full brick home (or both), and you are looking for furniture to fit into your federation home. Then, for example, if 'm' is a difficult sound for you, you could add that most furniture shops mainly stock mahogany type furniture whereas you are looking for more modern furniture.

It does not really matter if the content is a little strange. The important thing is to get as many of the difficult sounds into the dialogue as possible. This assignment could, of course, be done on the telephone or in a shop in person.

SUGGESTED HIERARCHY OF ASSIGNMENTS

We will start with the easiest assignment first, that is, number 10 at the bottom of the hierarchy list.

10. Ordering lunch

I always have trouble ordering salad sandwiches because of the 's' sounds. I would usually end up asking for a roll and specifying each ingredient when what I really wanted was a sandwich. The conversation used to go a little like this.

'Can I help you?'

'I'll have a . . . a . . . roll with . . . lettuce tomato . . . onion . . . carrot . . . beetroot . . .

'Are you asking me for a salad roll?'

'Yes.'

'Well, why didn't you say so?' And I would get a strange look.

So I started to do assignments ordering salad sandwiches. Armed with a tape-recorder you could go into your lunch shop and place an order using words you normally find difficult.

9. Having a conversation with a friend

This is an easy assignment. It is very simple when talking to a friend to introduce as many difficult words as possible into the conversation. I used to find saying people's names quite difficult, so during the conversation I used to try and mention as many friends by name as I could.

8. Talking to a friend on the telephone

This is essentially the same assignment as number 9 above, but you are talking on the telephone instead of face to face.

7. Telephoning a stranger

A good way to carry out this assignment is to ring up people who are selling something, for example, a secondhand car. Ask them all sorts of questions such as what colour it is, what mileage it's done, what model it is and so on.

Alternatively, you could telephone a store and ask questions about the goods that you wish to purchase. Use your imagination. I am sure you will come up with several interesting scenarios.

6. Making social introductions

Instead of avoiding making introductions (which you may have done in the past) actively seek them out. The next time you are invited to a social function, make a point of introducing a certain number of people to each other. Do a full introduction, that is, introduce each person using both their given name and their surname. You could increase the difficulty of the assignment, should the situation permit, by giving a little information about each person.

'Hello Tom. May I introduce Nick Tunbridge to you? Nick has recently returned from France where he was on holiday for two weeks.

Nick, this is Tom Cronin. Tom is a lawyer and is a partner in a law firm in the city.'

This is a very polite and pleasant way to introduce people and is excellent speech practice.

5. Making introductions at work

This is similar to the social occasion introduction, but as an assignment, it is a little more difficult. When you make the introduction try to expand it as much as possible. Introduce the most important person first, giving their name and position. Because this is a work-related introduction it is usually appropriate to give some background information on the person.

'Good morning Steve. May I introduce Joan King to you? Joan has recently joined the company as Region Sales Manager. Her background is in the photographics industry.'

Joan, this is Steve Dodds. Steve is our Marketing Director.'

Aim for these types of introductions in these assignments.

4. Conversing at work

This is number 4 on the hierarchy, so the situation would normally be a relatively stressful one. You could, for instance, try to talk to a difficult person or perhaps a very senior executive within the organisation, whom you would normally feel reluctant to enter into a conversation with.

The objectives of this assignment may vary. It may be that your main objective is to desensitise yourself. If this is the case, you may decide to use a voluntary stuttering technique. Alternatively, you may have as your objective fluent speech, in which case you may decide to use obvious technique and a slow rate of speech.

3. Telephoning at work

Make this assignment a difficult one. It is, after all, number 3 on the hierarchy. (Read 'The important phone call' in Chapter 7.)

I would suggest that you make a call to a senior executive of an important client company. Work out the objective of the assignment. In my case it would be a mixture of desensitising and fluency. I would be aiming for fluency, but using quite a lot of technique and speaking at around 180 spm.

2. Participating in a work meeting

Again, determine your objectives. Go into the meeting with the purpose of your assignment well in mind. (Don't forget to read Chapter 7 if the meeting is a hot spot for you.)

1. Making a presentation

I have covered the meeting and the presentation in other sections of this survival guide. The main thing to remember is to define your objective clearly and keep your mind on what you are trying to achieve. Don't forget to have your tape-recorder turned on.

Points to remember.
1. Work a hierarchy. You know your 'hot spots' better than anyone else.
2. Be creative and have fun with your assignments.
3. Be patient.
4. Be committed to achieving fluency.

CHAPTER SIX

FAMILY,
FRIENDS
AND
OTHERS

This chapter is for all the important people in your life — your wife, husband, parents, boyfriend, girlfriend, best friend — who do not stutter and who, for a long time, have accepted you as a stutterer. I encourage you to share this chapter with those who are close to you.

FAMILY AND FRIENDS

When I was undertaking treatment, the speech pathologists advised me not to expect to get a lot of recognition from my family regarding my new-found fluency. Take heart. This lack of comment is not a sign of indifference or rudeness. It is simply a sign that you are becoming like everybody else. You have just acquired the ability to speak with fluency. This ability may seem special to you but after a little while others may not even notice it.

When you arrive home after your treatment with your newly found fluency, you feel as though you're bringing home a new baby. Your new technique is fragile and it is dependent on your care and attention. You, of course, are overjoyed at having become a fluent speaker. You will be full of expectations about what you can achieve. Statistically though, you have very little chance of maintaining long-term fluency. You will need your family members to be there to help you through possibly the most difficult time in acquiring long-term fluency — the first three to six months after treatment.

The support structure so vital to your success will consist of speech buddies on one level and family and friends on another. They will need to monitor your progress carefully. They will need to watch for signs that you are not using your technique. They will need to push you into talking to your speech buddies if problems arise and persuade you to discuss your feelings with them, whether these feelings are positive or negative.

Here is an example of what form this support can take. Whenever my wife and I go out, my wife listens closely to my speech. If we are in a restaurant or at a friend's place for dinner and she feels that I am speaking too quickly or not using correct technique, she will give me a kick under the table. I still have the bruises! At the conclusion of the evening, or during it if there is a suitable moment, she will tell me what she thinks I am doing wrong. Her feedback is invaluable in helping me to keep on track.

Going from stuttering to speaking fluently is an enormous step. This change can affect more than just your speech. On particular occasions such as at parent/teacher meetings, your partner may be used to doing all the talking. You may find that this situation will change. Perhaps you will have to encourage it to change. If certain roles have been defined around your stutter, then when that stutter is removed, those roles may need to be redefined.

It is possible, after your course of treatment, that you will start speaking quickly with perfect fluency. You may not be interested in speaking slowly and using your technique. Encourage your family and friends to alert you to the dangers of spontaneous fluency.

Things will still go wrong. You will discover that stuttering and blocks will still occur. If you come home completely demoralised after a bad speech day, discuss the specific situation with your speech buddy and family. A bad day, or even several bad days, does not mean you are regressing. Learning to speak fluently with a technique is an evolving and growing exercise. The most important thing you must do after treatment is to try to carry out what you have been taught. If you make a mistake, learn from that mistake and try again. Every day is a new day. Learn this and apply it, not just to your speech, but to your life and I am sure you will succeed.

It is not an easy task for your partner to become a speech watchperson. Encourage them to understand how important it is to you to achieve your speech goal whether it is to be fluent or just to feel more comfortable about your speech. They will need to understand your technique so that they can watch for any signs of slipping. Work out an agreed signal so that they can gently remind you when they recognise that things are not going the way they should.

There is sometimes an interesting side effect when a stutterer gains a degree of fluency in their speech — depression! Sounds strange doesn't it? Why should some-one who has stuttered for so long and has finally achieved fluency become depressed about it? I think the answer is that when you stutter you can blame it for a lot of things. If you have always thought of yourself as having great potential and have regarded your stutter as the rope tied to your leg stopping you from rising in the world, you may get quite a shock when you realise that the rope is gone, but you are not rising! There may have been many factors preventing you from reaching your goals. Stuttering may or may not have been one of them.

You may realise that you are not as great as you believed and that your stutter may not have restricted you as much as you had thought. You may have to face the fact that perhaps you might not have as much talent as you thought.

My advice to your family and friends on how to handle this situation if it occurs, is to be gentle. Your family should talk to you about it. They should understand that a lifetime of stuttering is not just going to disappear without leaving some baggage behind. They should recognise that you are going through a period of adjustment. Remind them how much you hate stuttering and how much you want to overcome it. No matter what you think, getting rid of stuttering and speaking fluently is a major achievement and what the hell — your family and friends think you are great anyway!

They love you whether you stutter or not. They have proved that a thousand times. Their support will make a great difference not only to the maintenance of your fluency but also to your quality of life.

■ SPEAKING WITH FAMILY AND FRIENDS

Some stutterers find particular types of situations more difficult than do others. I have a friend who finds relaxing with his family a difficult situation. He claims he gets lazy and always ends up losing his technique and starts to stutter. I find relaxing with my family most comfortable for my speech, and I tend to 'normalise' in these situations.

A word of warning here. If you find speaking easier when you are with your family, take care that you do not let your technique slip. Even though you feel in control, you must still maintain your technique. After I had completed treatment, I found it very tempting to ease my level of concentration in situations where I felt I had a lot of control over my speech, such as weekends at home with my wife. Away from the pressures of the office, I could speed up to around 240 spm and stay perfectly fluent.

That was fine until Monday morning came around. I was so used to the two days speaking at 240 spm using a low level of technique and attaining high 'normalisation' that I found it really difficult making the adjustment to the use of the high level of technique I needed to get through the day at work.

Be very careful not to allow yourself to 'normalise' to such a degree that you feel uncomfortable about reverting back to an obvious level of technique if required.

You may or may not be comfortable about changing your particular role in the family, but it will be in your interest that you learn to become more vocal and start to carry your share of 'speaking duties'. It is important for your family to help you to accept this change and encourage you to become as much of a voice for the family as you really wish to be.

PEOPLE'S REACTIONS TO STUTTERERS

I have based this section on my own experiences and what I consider would have been of benefit to me as a stutterer. Your situation may be entirely different and may call for different reactions, but nevertheless my experiences may provide fluent-speaking people with some insight into how to relate to stutterers.

All my stuttering life I was confused about what my listeners felt when I was stuttering. When I was about 14 I had, for some reason or other, to visit the local police station. I remember this visit very clearly. There was an unusual amount of activity at the station this day and a lot of uniformed and plain-clothed policemen were running about. I was looking for someone who could tell me where to find the person I had come to see.

The policeman who asked me what I wanted was a very large detective who seemed to be about three times my size. He had to bend forward to try and hear me when I spoke. But I didn't speak. I was so utterly intimidated I suffered a severe block. I tried to speak, but no words came — just a series of noises as I breathed deeply and gasped and breathed and gasped. Then I discovered that this giant of a man was in a state of total shock. The poor guy was so embarrassed he didn't know where to look. I took in this picture and thought that if I had this effect on a seasoned cop, how on earth did I appear to other people when I stuttered? I have long forgotten why I was at the station, but I shall never forget the policeman's reaction to my block.

What do non-stutterers go through when we stutterers have our little moments? It is probably not easy to be the listener.

Most people when confronted by a stutterer who is experiencing difficulty speaking, will finish the word or sentence for them. This may be annoying to the stutterer, but it is a normal reaction. Some people will adopt a kind of trance-like look and pretend that nothing unusual is happening. Other listeners get so embarrassed they laugh, or look at the sky or stare at their shoes. Again, quite normal reactions. Sometimes the listener just walks away from the speaker and the situation. I know. It's happened to me. I feel sorry for the kind of person who can only cope with a difficult situation by walking away from it.

■ PUT YOURSELF IN THE STUTTERER'S SHOES

The first thing to do is to think about your reaction to the stutterer. Stuttering has nothing to do with a mental disorder. Stutterers are just as mentally alert as their listeners. They are aware of your reaction to them. It is said that the spoken word represents about 35% of total communication. It is a very important 35%, particularly when as a stutterer you do not have full access to it.

You do not stutter. Think about how you would feel if your job depended on your speaking articulately. How much of your self-esteem rests on your ability to impress people by your speech? What value do you place on first impressions, that first couple of minutes when you assess people by the way they look and the way they speak?

How would you fare in society today if you were unable to speak the way you do? How would you feel if you were unable to say your own name without a major physical and emotional effort? Then think of the stutterer with a bright agile mind, trying to speak. It is like a car with a V8 engine and no wheels. It can make a lot of noise, but it can't go anywhere.

You, as a 'normal' speaker, can make a successful career for yourself in any field you choose. Think of the stutterers who quite often find themselves employed in positions beneath their abilities because they choose a job that enables them to hide away from the normal demands of communication.

So the next time you meet a stutterer who is having difficulty with their speech, think of how you would cope if you stuttered and how you would like to be treated. In my opinion, the best listeners show patience and under-standing. If the stutterer is having extreme difficulty, ask them if they mind if you helped. If they indicate that they do not mind, then say the word or phrase for them. Do not presume though, that they want you to finish all their sentences for them. And what of the complaint that listening to a stutterer takes too much time? How busy is your life that you cannot spare a little extra time for another human being who wants to communicate with you? You only have to listen to this person for a brief moment. They have to live with their stutter 24 hours a day.

IF YOUR CHILD STUTTERS

There are several things you can do to help if you have a child who stutters. You can:

- give support
- have patience
- encourage them to talk to speech buddies
- stop feeling guilty over the situation.

Give support

I suggest that you seek help immediately, to prevent your child developing behavioural characteristics that may be counterproductive to future therapy. Many people believe it is natural for children to stutter and believe they will grow out of this. Current thought by speech pathologists and psychologists is that it is not worth the risk to hesitate obtaining professional treatment for your child.

When your child has a bad stuttering bout or a complete block, do not remind them that they are not speaking well. They know this themselves! Choose an appropriate moment and try to find out how you can help.

Build up a support structure for your child. Your support as parents and the support of speech buddies, together with your patience and love, are the things that will help your child build up their self-confidence.

Be patient
If your child is entering their teens, they will be having difficulties coping with physical changes as well as coming to terms with their speech difficulties. Do not get impatient with them for stuttering. If they have had therapy and are not using their technique properly, try to determine why. Keep the channels of communication open as much as you can. This may not be easy, particularly if your child is trying to deal with the stutter by not talking.

Encourage them to talk to speech buddies
It is very important for your child to have friends who also stutter and who have had treatment for it. These friends will become part of their support group and may be there all the way through your child's life, or at least their school life.

Don't feel guilty
Under no circumstances look at your child with guilt in your eyes, blaming yourself for their stutter. Most research now seems to suggest that stuttering is genetic. You did not plan to produce a child that stuttered. It was just the way things worked out. It is not your fault that your child stutters. Try to make their life as easy as possible and make them feel good about their home life. Concentrate on these positive aspects and not on blame. Later on, when they

are adults, they will look back on their childhood and remember the love and support their parents gave them.

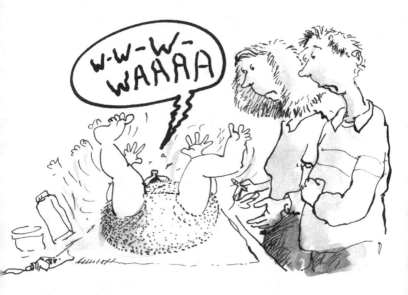

CHAPTER SEVEN

HOT

SPOTS

We all find ourselves from time to time in certain situations that we would prefer to avoid. I call these situations 'hot spots'. For me, they typically involve speaking at some sort of formal occasion. My record of speaking on formal occasions is not good, so I tend not to look forward to these events.

Since learning my technique, however, I have approached these hot spots in a way that has minimised my chance of stuttering and, as a result, I have changed my attitude towards many speaking situations. I no longer consider packing my bags and heading for the hills should such hot spot occasions arise. I now approach all hot spots in a way that usually guarantees a successful speaking result. In this chapter I describe hot spot situations and what you can do to get through them.

SCHOOLDAYS

I remember these days well. Looking back I find it incredible that I stuttered my way through all the levels of my education. Dealing with normal adolescent development, as well as with class and social situations, was a lot to handle without the added problem of a stutter.

I still remember at high school trying to save face whilst stuttering in front of the class when delivering a presentation. Unfortunately students usually have not yet developed mature social skills, and someone stuttering brings shouts from the class of 'sit down' and 'get someone who can talk'. Not exactly subtle.

I did not like stuttering and I dreamed of becoming perfectly fluent. In those days I loved to watch Perry Mason. It was my dream to become a barrister. I imagined myself making the same wonderful courtroom appearances that Perry Mason did.

Alongside the dream, however, was the nightmare. I saw myself in court, not as the silver-tongued Perry Mason, but as the stuttering Nick Tunbridge. I was always representing the same man, a man falsely accused of murder. His only salvation lay in the hands of his barrister. You've guessed what happened. I stood up and delivered a speech for the defence so riddled with stutters that no jury would ever believe me when I pleaded that the accused was innocent. I decided it was too big a risk — both for myself and future clients — to pursue my dream of becoming a barrister.

It might be a bit daunting to think of pleading on someone's behalf in the courtroom, but by practising your speech and following your technique, you should be able to speak competently in most of the troublesome situations you will encounter during your school career. I am basing my suggestions on the problems I remember having. I am presuming that you have learned your technique and that you have had, or are currently undertaking, some kind of speech therapy.

For me, there were five main problem areas:
1. answering questions in class
2. asking questions in class
3. reading aloud in class
4. giving a presentation in class
5. going to parties.

■ ANSWERING QUESTIONS

I remember when I was about 16 sitting in a mathematics class on a bright sunny Australian day. The term had only just started and we had finished a test designed to enable the teacher to assess which students had an aptitude for mathematics. The teacher went through the roll asking each student to call out their marks.

I was nervous about this. My mark was 44 out of 50 and I had difficulty pronouncing 'f' sounds. You can imagine how delighted I was with my result! As my name came closer, I started to panic. To calm myself I started chattering nervously to the student sitting next to me and then the inevitable happened. I heard my name yelled out.

I stood up to say 'forty-four' but nothing happened. I tried harder to get the words out. Still nothing. Finally, a slight 'f' sound emerged and after stuttering, the rest of the word followed. The whole class was in shock. The teacher was in shock. I was exhausted. Then the teacher spoke, 'Tunbridge, I just wanted you to stop talking. We

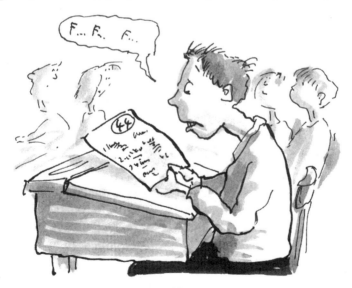

are not up to you yet!' And I had to sit while names were called, waiting to hear mine and knowing I had the whole process to go through again.

What had happened here? Firstly, I had no technique to call on. I had not yet been taught a technique. Secondly, I had let the fear of trying to say a problem sound grow to such a stage that I had no option but to stutter.

Now let's put you in that classroom, but armed with your technique.

Do not panic. Have confidence in your technique. As your name comes closer, concentrate on your technique and in your mind repeat to yourself the words that you are going to say. When the teacher calls your name, keep calm, use your technique and simply say out loud what you were saying to yourself. Remember to speak slowly and use your technique.

When you answer a question, whether voluntarily or whether required to, you must never forget your technique and the skills at your disposal. As a suggestion, follow this plan.

- *Do not answer immediately.* Wait a few seconds. The pause will help your delivery anyway.
- *Desensitise yourself.* It does not matter how you sound. If your technique is to start speaking very slowly then that is precisely what you should do.

You need to cultivate your technique and your school friends are just going to have to accept that you are doing this to overcome your stutter. You need to face the fact that you have a lifetime of speaking situations and you need to get over any feelings of embarrassment. (See Chapter 3 on desensitising.)

■ ASKING QUESTIONS

Have you ever been in the situation in which you have a question you really want to ask, but you just can't get the words out? I suppose everyone has. I remember listening to a lecture and realising the lecturer had not covered a particular issue. There was a question that I really wanted to ask. I put my hand up and then very quickly put it down again because I knew I would probably stutter when asking the question. It would be safer to ask the lecturer later on.

It's time to stop your stutter rearing its head and interrupting your pursuit of knowledge. Here's the plan.

- *Write the question out.* When a question comes into your mind as you are listening to the lecture, jot it down. It does not have to be in full. Note form will do.
- *Read the question.* You have the written note of your question in front of you. Transfer it from the paper to your 'mind screen' and visualise the words before you say them, using whatever level of technique is necessary. Do not let your fear of stuttering stop you from asking your question. Use your technique and stay fluent.

■ READING ALOUD

The most important thing to remember about reading aloud in class is **not to be rushed**. It is very easy to speed up in this situation. Read slowly and concentrate on your technique.

If there is any discussion prior to the reading or the opportunity to ask questions, I suggest that you do so, this way you can 'warm up' a little. While reading, pause a lot. This has two beneficial effects. Firstly, it slows you down, and allows you to concentrate on your reading. Secondly, it adds colour to what you are reading.

For example, I recently had to undertake some training for my job in a situation very similar to that of the classroom. Each person in the group of about 15 people had a textbook to work from, and the trainer asked various people to read certain passages aloud. I found that although I had been in the workforce for over 12 years, I was going through the same fears I had had when I was at school. The guy next to me, who worked in a senior position at a bank, was reading aloud very quickly. This did not help my fear at all. I thought to myself, 'I can't talk slowly. I can't use my technique in this situation. I am going to stutter.'

At that moment my positive thoughts took over from the negative. I remembered the desensitising I had done and all the hard work I had put in to get to where I was today. When the trainer eventually asked me to read, I was ready. I paused. There was a long silence as I took the time needed to get myself ready. And I read slowly. Not only did I *not* stutter, but in my opinion I read better than most of the others in the group — better because I read clearly and at a pace that I considered was easy to listen to.

Reading aloud at school is not easy, but you can do it. Do it in your own time, in your own way, and do not listen to anyone.

■ GIVING A PRESENTATION

At school there was a wonderful subject called English Expression. I loved it. I loved it because I could stand in front of the class and take on another identity. As you've guessed, I was fluent when I spoke.

I remember the first 'acting performance' I gave to the bemused students of my English Expression class. I recited the poem, *Jabberwocky*, by Lewis Carroll. I got up in front of the class and almost as if by divine blessing, as long as I was in full 'theatrics', I did not stutter. It felt wonderful. I moved from reciting poems to acting scenarios from short plays that I had written. This 'fluency' was short lived and really required the novelty of a different persona to enable it to survive. This is not a practical method of attaining fluency. The use of a more 'suitable' technique is a better option.

Throughout life you will have to give presentations of one sort or another. They start at school and continue throughout your life. Whether the occasion is work-related or social, you will have to give some kind of presentation or speech at some stage.

If you have to give a presentation to your school class, read the material on 'giving presentations' later in this chapter. It sounds as though there's a lot of effort involved, but it works for me and I hope it will be of benefit to you. Give it a try. You have nothing to lose and everything to gain.

■ PARTIES

Coping with social situations while you are at school or college can be a problem if you stutter, particularly if it involves meeting new people. It is easy to get nervous and really blow it. What I would suggest is that before you go to the party, you work out some sort of plan.

You have to remember to keep using your technique. This will mean you have to keep concentrating on your speech. In a party atmosphere that is not going to be easy, especially if you tend to talk faster as you become more involved in the party. You will have to drop your speech rate down to a much slower level and treat the evening as a good desensitising assignment. If that is just not possible, then use enough technique to at least get you through the evening.

There will be many situations in your life in which you will be tempted to drop your technique. You should get into good habits now, and resist this temptation. Don't let your friends influence the way you speak. It's you who has the stutter, and you who has learned a technique to overcome it.

When schooldays are over, your friends will go off on their chosen career paths. You will follow your own path. The chances are that your stutter will still be there with you. This is why it is very important that you learn how to deal with it as early as possible. Do whatever you can to reinforce your technique. Do not be concerned if your friends think you sound strange when you talk.

And don't forget to enjoy the party.

■ ENJOYING YOUR SCHOOLDAYS

It can be daunting at school to think that you still have a long time ahead of you fighting your stutter. Take heart. At least today people have a fighting chance of attaining fluency.

Doors will open and close for you all through your life. You have a stutter and have to face that fact. But you do not have to face it on your own. You should involve sympathetic people whom you feel can help you. Get as much help and support as you can.

And one more thing. Don't worry too much about your speech. There are a lot of really good times to be had during your schooldays. Don't let your speech interfere with your enjoyment. Work on your speech, try to control it as best you can, don't close people out of your life and above all, have a good time!

AT WORK

■ MAKING INTRODUCTIONS

This used to be one of the situations I feared most, whether it was a social or a work-related occasion. I would lie awake worrying about the forthcoming introduction. I would practise it in my mind over and over again. What I saw in my mind's eye was an image of myself stuttering uncontrollably whilst the people stared at me in alarm and then went about introducing themselves.

The fear
Let's look at the fear of stuttering during the introduction.

An occasion is looming on the horizon at which you have to introduce people. You are afraid because you always have difficulty in doing this. Your fear is increased both because there will be people present who do not know you are a stutterer, and because the thought of stuttering in front of anybody scares you.

Why are you so afraid of making introductions? What is the worst thing that can happen? If the situation is a social one, the worst thing is that you will be embarrassed. But your stutter has embarrassed you before and if you continue to stutter it will certainly embarrass you in the future. So, this is just another of those embarrassing moments. Your fear of embarrassment feeds on itself and grows very rapidly. Don't let it grow.

What is the worst possible thing that can happen in a work-related situation? Are you likely to get fired if you stutter badly whilst introducing someone? I doubt it very much and quite frankly, if you did, then I think your job was very shaky to begin with. Let's design a plan so that we minimise the chance of stuttering.

Minimising the fear

Firstly, it is absolutely imperative that you block out as much fear about the forthcoming occasion as you can. If you can't overcome it, then you have to summon up the courage to carry on regardless. We only fear situations we feel we have no control over. This is understandable, particularly if you have not had sufficient record of success in making introductions without stuttering and you consequently keep telling yourself that you will stutter. Although it's difficult, you have to stop thinking like a stutterer. You have to think that you have a skill, although newly developing, that gives you control over your speech.

Controlling the stutter

You are still learning to control your stutter. You mightn't be able to give a speech at 270 spm. But you can speak *in full control* and handle an introduction by using your technique and speaking at 180–200 spm. Remember, if you stutter it is because you have chosen, consciously or unconsciously, not to use your technique. The deciding point will be how desensitised you are. If you have become sufficiently desensitised, you will use the technique and *not* stutter. This will give you the bonus of adding another success to your record, so the next time you have to perform introductions you will have the thought of this win to call on. If you are still self-conscious about how you sound, you most probably will choose not to use your technique and will stutter.

Planning the introduction

Here's the scenario. You are an account executive and at a meeting, you have to introduce the senior management of your company to the senior management of the client company. The meeting is to take place at the client's premises and the introductions will occur after everybody is seated. You have to introduce people by name and position. This sounds terrifying.

If you have come to terms with your fear, you will probably do well. If you haven't, pull yourself together and realise that you will be more critical of your performance than anyone else will. Relax, and tell yourself you can do the introductions successfully.

Walk into the room and take your seat. The first thing you have to do is make a decision. Are you going to speak at 180–200 spm and think about what you are doing or are you going to blurt out the introduction at your normal speed and hope to make it?

If you have decided to speak slowly and use your technique, set your pace by saying your first few words very slowly, at say, 150–180 spm. Then increase the rate slowly up to the 200 spm as the introductions proceed. Remember to pause and to breathe properly. If you forget your technique momentarily and start feeling tense, just stop, breathe and start again.

To perform the introductions well, you really have to become desensitised. Remember that your only other option is to risk stuttering. The more successful you are on occasions like these, the closer you are to being in control of your speech.

■ SPEAKING AT A MEETING

Everybody attends meetings at some stage of their lives. Although I think the majority of meetings take place in the work environment, other types of meetings can provide challenges. There are parent/teacher meetings, religious meetings, social club meetings, sports club meetings, committee meetings and many, many others. No matter what sort of meeting you are intending to speak at, you need to prepare for it.

Anxiety or stress usually occurs because you do not have a good grasp of the subject matter you are presenting. Researching your subject will reduce your level of anxiety, thus enabling you to be in total control during the meeting. This sounds great in theory but how can it be achieved?

Preparing for the sales meeting

Firstly, know exactly what you want to say and then practise your speech preferably no later than one hour beforehand. I suggest that you divide your practice session into two. Spend 50% of your practice session with a speech buddy and for the other 50%, choose a work colleague. Practise talking at the speed that you intend to speak at during the meeting. The work colleague you are talking to should not know you are practising. During the session, use as many of the relevant terms as you can. This way, you will be ready for the meeting and will not go into a potentially difficult situation cold.

Secondly, avoid doing anything that is likely to add to your nervousness, such as drinking coffee, smoking, etc. Drink water if you are thirsty and relax. Close your eyes for a couple of minutes and repeat some positive statements to yourself, such as 'I have the technique not to stutter' and 'I have control over my speech'. When the meeting starts, stay relaxed. Remember to breathe properly and whenever you speak, stay true to your practice with your speech buddy. The more success you have using your technique, the easier the meetings become.

Preparing for the social club meeting

In a moment of unbridled enthusiasm, you have offered to be treasurer for your son's football club and you have to present the financial statement at the next meeting. Since you know beforehand exactly what you will be saying, this presents fewer problems than if your role is not so exactly defined.

As for any meeting:
- know your subject
- write out exactly what you will be saying
- identify the troublesome words. Take special care over any numbers that you find particularly difficult to say
- get your speech buddy on the phone and practise what you have to say
- then role-play your part of the meeting. This will give you confidence and will certainly reduce your overall fear of the situation.

If you are attending the meeting with your partner or a

friend or, even better, with a speech buddy, work out a sign they can make if they think you are straying from your technique.

■ THE INTERVIEW

You are looking good! The new dark blue suit says it all; your shoes are polished; you look like a million dollars on a sunny day. You are going to go into that interview and you are going to get that job!

Hold it right there! You've got some speech work to do. This interview is going to be so important to your future that you must prepare for it. This must be done well before the interview. You have to feel absolutely confident about your speech. You cannot be preoccupied about whether you will stutter or not. Your only thought for your speech should be on your technique. This means that you can concentrate on answering questions and performing well at the interview.

The rehearsal

At least two or three days before the interview get together with a speech buddy and tell them about the forthcoming interview. Next, write out everything you want to say, then rehearse it with your speech buddy. Get your speech buddy to listen to you and evaluate your performance. By practising with him or her you will be prepared for questions you may be asked and by rehearsing thoroughly, you should perform well in all areas at the interview.

Determine the rate that you want to speak at. Become familiar with it so that if you start to speed up you will be aware of it. The more often you have rehearsed and the more material you have committed to memory, the less likely you are to focus on troublesome words and become panicky. If you do not practise and rehearse what you are going to say, you may tend to worry about words that cause you difficulty.

In the interview you are practically certain to be asked the name of your current employer. If, for instance, you work at Sammy Seal's Supermarket and have trouble with 's' words, you may concentrate on trying to work out when these words are likely to come up in the conversation and be figuring out how to avoid saying them.

You must be able to concentrate on the conversation, not on stuttering. You cannot risk taking your mind off what is being said at the interview. If you practise beforehand, a 'Sammy Seals' block as depicted in the following cartoon will probably not occur.

A speech reminder

When you go into the interview you will be carrying a briefcase or perhaps a folder. I put a little yellow sticker onto the folder and every time I look at it during the interview I remember why I put it there and what it represents. It represents my speech. It reminds me that speaking well is the most important thing I can do at the interview. My objective is to maintain fluency with correct use of my technique. The sticker also reminds me of all the work I have done in preparing for this interview.

I strongly suggest that you follow this advice prior to interviews. I have found it to be very successful and I am sure you agree that you are going to significantly increase your chances of getting that new job if you can speak fluently at the interview.

THE INTERVIEW

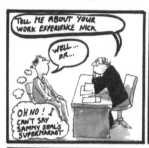

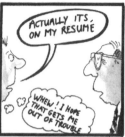

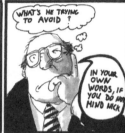

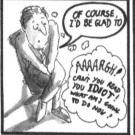

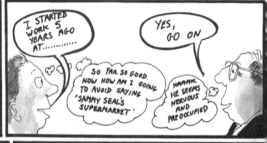

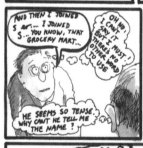

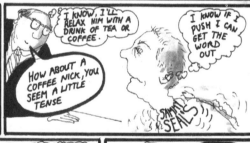

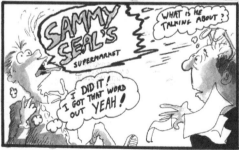

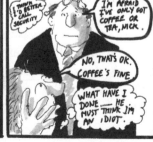

■ THE IMPORTANT PHONE CALL

What forms your worst nightmare? I have this horrible vision. It sits with a stillness that can only be described as deathly. Its body is like no other. It is fat with a repulsive gridlike face and a huge twisted tail. The creature screams like a thousand high pitched bells. And it is always screaming my name. Well, maybe the phone does not appear exactly like that to you, but I think it's a safe bet that every stutterer has special hate feelings for the phone.

However much we stutterers might like to abolish the phone, it is here to stay. Most people use it every day. In some occupations, you can spend the majority of your time telephoning. These are the sorts of things that can occur during your day at work.

THE PLANNED OFFICE CALL

You are a salesperson and you have to call the manager of a company. Now let's make it difficult! Let us assume that this manager is a friend of the manager of the company that you work for, so you know that your phone call will be relayed back to your manager. To make matters more difficult, the manager that you are calling hates your products and does not want to hear from you. He is taking the call only because of his friendship with your manager. The call has been arranged for a predetermined time, say 10.30 am. Here is what you have to decide.

What do you want to achieve by making this phone call? Several things. You want to create a good impression. You want the manager of the other company to see you as a knowledgeable and articulate person. You want to persuade him that your company's products are worth

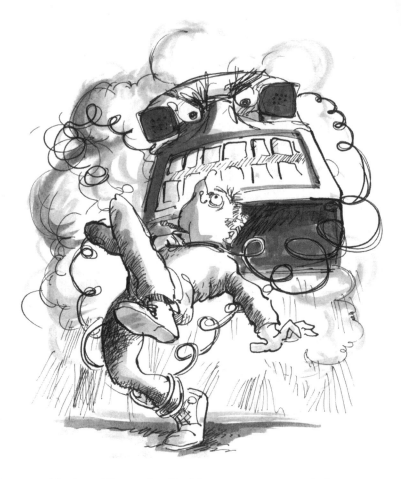

considering. Through all this you want to reinforce your worth to your own company.

Your plan must take into account the following:
1. The need to make a good impression.
2. The need to achieve fluent speech.

Unless you talk fluently, you may run the risk of not making a good impression. So you need to draw up your plan carefully in order to reach both goals.

1. Making a good impression
I would suggest that you prepare in-depth for the call.

- Work out the questions the manager is likely to ask and have all the answers ready.
- Learn everything you can about the person you are calling.
- Find out about their company's needs.
- Know every last detail about your own product.

The more confident you are about your call, the less stress you are likely to feel and, of course, the less stress you feel, the less likely you are to abandon your technique and risk stuttering.

2. Attaining fluent speech
(a) Write out the full text of the intended conversation.
Make a list of any words you know you have difficulty with. Practise saying them so that you become very familiar with them. This reduces the risk of panicking and resorting to word avoidance. Have the text in front of you when you make the call.

By becoming familiar with the full text, you may avoid unpleasant surprises. It also means that you sound as though you know your subject really well.

(b) Practise the text with your speech buddy.
The second step is to practise your speech with one of your patient speech buddies. Go over it and over it, the night before if possible. Your familiarity with it will mean you have a positive attitude towards the text. When the time comes to actually make the call, you know that you have already spoken the words half a dozen times at least, with perfect fluency.

Another advantage of practising the telephone call several times with a speech buddy is that when you are talking to the general manager, you can make yourself feel more relaxed by closing your eyes and imagining you are talking to your speech buddy. I have found this really helps!

(c) Make the hierarchy of calls.

On the morning of your call, build up to it in a controlled way by making a hierarchy of calls. Start by practising with your speech buddy and then make four other calls. The first should be an easy one, say to a friend. The fourth should be a more demanding — but relatively safe call. You could, for example, call a colleague and discuss something work-related. Record your part in these calls on your tape-recorder. You will need to play some of these back to your speech buddy for evaluation prior to making the 'real' call. During these four hierarchy calls, be on the lookout for 'cracks' in your technique and pay strict attention to your speed.

(d) Practise.

The purpose of calling your speech buddy is to practise your conversation 15 minutes before you make your first hierarchy call. Make sure you are practising with the same speech buddy that you ran through the text with on the previous night. The purpose of this 15 minute practice is to get you focussed so that you can make sure that your technique is working.

After you have finished the hierarchy calls, get back on the phone to your speech buddy for another 15 minutes of practice. Play back some of the recorded hierarchy of calls so that your speech buddy can offer criticism. Ask your speech buddy to identify any area of weakness.

(e) Make the important call.
It's 10.30 and you are ready to make the call. Put the text in front of you, and turn your tape-recorder on. Both these actions will remind you of all the preparation you have done.

(f) Evaluate your performance.
After you have made the important company call, talk to your speech buddy. Play the taped recording so that you can both evaluate your side of the conversation.

Preparing for important calls like this one is a lot of work. But using the system I describe can mean the difference between failure and success for those important 'career' phone calls. It is worth the effort to make sure you maximise your control over your conversations rather than leaving things to chance.

There is a second benefit in preparing thoroughly in this way. If you find that you can start to make pressurised calls like this fluently, you will really start to replace negative experiences with positive. The overall effect of this on your fluency maintenance is great, believe me!

ANSWERING THE UNEXPECTED CALL

The procedure outlined only works for prearranged calls. What do you do when you do not get advance warning about the call and have to make it immediately?

This is not an easy situation. You have had no warning and there is no time to organise to practise with your speech buddy. Your success in this situation will come down to how desensitised you are. The situation puts you under pressure and there will be additional pressure if your manager happens to be in the office and wants to listen to the call.

Firstly, you have to make a decision. Is fluent speech your first priority? The answer to this should be 'yes'. If you answer 'no', I believe you will stutter during your telephone conversation. Using your technique means your speech will not sound perfectly normal but, let's face it, you are *not* a normal speaker. At least you will be speaking fluently. If you don't use your technique you risk blundering your way through with word avoidance and stuttering. If you *do* use word avoidance, you run another risk. You may not be able to express yourself in the exact way you wish. This may result in both managers — the one on the phone and the one in front of you — getting the wrong idea about your abilities.

This is how to deal with the situation if you are aiming for fluency.

Step 1
Slow right down. Even if you think you sound like a moron, speak slowly to retain control over your words. No-one has lost a job for talking too slowly. Do not worry about what the listeners will think. The chances are they will not even notice. Even if they do, they will probably not comment.

Step 2
Try and tape your speech. I carry my tape-recorder with me at all times in my jacket or shirt pocket. If you manage to tape your part of the conversation, it will provide you with a valuable record of how you sound under pressure.

Also, knowing that the tape is on will help keep your mind on your technique.

Step 3
If you feel tense, be prepared to use your technique in its strongest form. Forget about who else is listening. Imagine you are in a room full of speech buddies. This sort of call is not easy for anyone and how you succeed will depend on how proficient you are at your technique and how desensitised you are to using it.

If you manage well in a situation as pressured as this, then pat yourself on the back. Not only will you have had a positive experience, but you will have gone a long way towards becoming desensitised.

■ THE PRESENTATION

(a) List your priorities.
Priorities in making a presentation are:
- to be fluent
- to present material worth listening to.

Both priorities are equally important to you. Listing your priorities gives you the areas within your preparation to focus on and keeps you moving in the right direction.

(b) Write out your presentation.
Write out the material you are presenting. The best way to do this is to write out a couple of paragraphs at a time, then say them as if you were presenting them. Write out instructions to yourself also. For example, if you want to pause at a particular time and refer to a visual aid to stress a point, make a note of that action and memorise where it will occur.

The purpose of writing out the presentation is so that everything is well thought through and planned. Look on your presentation as a performance. Your written words and the notes of your actions form your script.

(c) Memorise your presentation.
You must become completely familiar with your talk so that you can reduce the tension sufficiently to ensure that you use your technique and can concentrate on your fluency. In order to do this you must know exactly what you are going to say and that means committing it to memory. The words and actions must be so well learned that they become second nature to you.

(d) Use visual aids.
Visual aids are good devices to use. They help stress a point and they make the presentation more interesting. You can refer to a slide, point to it and discuss it. People will turn their attention to the image on the wall which will give you a bit of a breather.

(e) Research your questions and answers.
If possible, try and prepare answers for most of the questions you are likely to be asked. Obviously you will not be prepared for *all* the questions, but you will have a reasonable idea of most of the ones you are likely to be faced with. Prepare the answers for those. The better you prepare, the more relaxed you will become.

Should someone ask a difficult question that you are unprepared for and you find it has thrown you 'off balance', slip down to a slower speech rate and put a little more technique into your speech.

(f) Practise with speech buddies.
Get together with as many speech buddies as you can. The objective here is to do a rehearsal of the presentation with a group of people who can really evaluate your use of technique. Try to get together with at least four speech buddies and go through the entire presentation as you will do it on the day. By now, of course, you have committed it to memory. Listen carefully to their evaluation.

It is also a good idea to tape this rehearsal so that you can listen to it later and hear any mistakes you are making.

(g) Practise with friends/relatives.
This rehearsal is a little less speech-friendly than the previous rehearsal with your speech buddies.

Your friends or relatives will probably evaluate your performance less critically than your speech buddies — certainly as far as your fluency goes. But I think you will find that this rehearsal is more nerve-wracking than the one with your speech buddies. Make sure that you tape this session and watch your speed.

(h) Rehearse with work colleagues.
This rehearsal is the last hurdle to leap before the event. Everything that you do and say during this rehearsal should be exactly the same as during the actual presentation. The aim of this rehearsal is to reduce your stress about the situation and to assist you with your desensitisation on the day.

I suggest you ignore whatever feedback your work colleagues give you regarding your speech. If they say you should speak faster or with less technique tell them that you cannot. Your level of technique and speed by this stage are set. What they hear now is what they are going to get on the day.

You have written your presentation out. You have committed it to memory. You have practised it so many times that you are completely familiar with it. Your speech buddies have heard it, your family and friends have heard it, and your work colleagues have heard it. There are no surprises left to encounter. The nerves that you feel about the situation are the normal stage nerves that most people feel before any public speaking situation. They are not stutterers' nerves. You have done more than enough preparation. Remember all the elements of your technique and watch your speed at all times. Turn on your pocket tape-recorder and go out there and give a great presentation. You have worked hard and you deserve your success.

■ CLIENT MEETING WITH COLLEAGUE/MANAGER

Perhaps you are totally comfortable calling on a client on your own. However, it is a totally different matter if you have to take a colleague with you or, even worse, if your boss comes along for the ride. Then you are likely to fall into a heap. Why does this happen?

I believe there are two reasons.

1. You may be unprepared. When you are alone with the client you do not feel that there is anyone to question your knowledge of your subject. This gives you confidence. Having someone else there who also knows the subject can put you off.

2. You are not desensitised sufficiently with your colleagues or manager. You need to overcome any inferiority feelings you have. You may feel you are not

as good at your work as this person, because they are fluent and you stutter. You have your technique, use it.

I suggest that you follow this plan of action.

- Firstly, prepare for the client visit. You should be doing this anyway, whether you stutter or not. Know your subject matter backwards. Know the answers to any possible questions. This will make you feel more relaxed about having an audience.

- Secondly, desensitise yourself with your colleague or manager. Client visits such as these are rarely surprise visits. You will probably have known about it in advance. Practise your technique with your colleague or colleagues prior to the client visit to desensitise yourself.

- Thirdly, do not worry about what your colleagues or manager may think of the way you sound. It is of no importance. You are being paid to do a job, and by using your technique, you are speaking in the best way you can.

Forget about their perceptions, and concentrate on the client visit.

IMPORTANT SOCIAL MOMENTS

I would define as an important social moment any occasion that requires you to give a speech. The social occasion may be a birthday, a wedding, a retirement party. Perhaps one of the most important events would be your own wedding when, as the groom, you will have to make a speech at the reception or, at the very least, say 'I do'. There are many other important types of social situations.

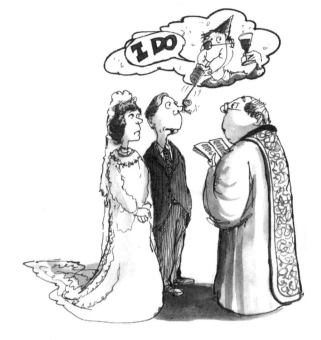

When called on to speak on one of these occasions, you can develop a plan to minimise the risk of stuttering.

- Have a positive attitude.
- Do your preparation.

Have a positive attitude

It is important that you have your attitude clearly defined. Do not have these situations marred by a feeling of disappointment because you stuttered. It is most important that you look back with a feeling of joy on what was a wonderful occasion, not with disappointment because it was a poor speech situation for you. Hopefully you will not stutter, but if you do, do not worry. Nobody will care about your stuttering as much as you do, so just relax.

Relaxing does not mean you can let your technique slip. The plan is to be as fluent as you can. Your attitude to the occasion should be well thought out and positive. Most social events that call for a speech are usually a celebration of some kind — so celebrate! Enjoy yourself. Do not let fear mar your enjoyment. You have been called upon to give a speech because your friends want to hear what you have to say. Any fear you feel can be reduced by preparation.

Prepare for the event
Treat this event in the same way as any other public speaking task.
1. Write out your text.
2. Commit it to memory.
3. Rehearse with your speech buddy.
4. Rehearse with people other than your speech buddy.
5. Make your speech.
I have covered the above steps in detail earlier in the chapter. The more prepared you are, the less likely you will be to stutter.

A word of warning
If the social event you have to give a speech at is a party, I want to sound a word of warning. Try not to enjoy it too much — you know what I mean! Alcohol and technique do not usually go well together. I have some friends who stutter and who tell me it does not cause them any trouble. I think it is better to play it safe. I always make sure I have my feet firmly on the ground before I have to perform any function at a social event. I would suggest that you maintain that attitude right through the evening. That way you will ensure that you minimise your chance of stuttering.

COPING WITH STRESS, ILLNESS AND FATIGUE

There are times when your technique may not work. After all, we are humans, not machines! When you feel stress or fatigue or are ill, you may find that your speech will let you down.

■ COPING WITH STRESS

Avoid stress if you possibly can. In the top drawer of my desk at work I have a plastic card which is called a stress monitor. When you place your thumb on a little pad, this device reads the temperature of your thumb and this triggers a colour change around the pad. The colour change indicates whether you are calm or tense, alert, relaxed or stressed. I have been amazed how accurate this device can be in alerting me to how I am feeling. I have used it during phone calls and I have found it particularly enlightening.

When you are feeling stress there is a good chance it will affect your performance negatively in all areas. I believe that most stress is caused by two factors:

- Firstly, when you feel that the expectation placed on you by others is undeliverable.
- Secondly, when events that affect your performance are outside your control.

I will explain what I mean here by relating it to a work situation. If you are expected to have knowledge of a certain subject and you do not, or if you are expected to have completed work on something by a certain date and are running late, you will feel stress. This situation is manageable. It requires preparation or time management skills to ensure that all the work or information is to hand at the required time. If, however, your computer breaks down and you need it to complete this work, there is nothing you can do about it. This situation will most probably cause you stress because the circumstances are outside your control.

I have found it helpful to be aware of my stress levels. When I feel stressed I try to analyse why I am feeling this way and work out what I can do to remove or reduce the stress. Monitoring your stress level and trying to control it will probably benefit you in all areas of your life and not just in your speech.

Stuttering causes stress

Every stutterer knows that stuttering itself leads to feelings of stress. Before acquiring a technique, you were living with a kind of time bomb. Some days your speech would be quite fluent, other days you would stutter badly and there appeared to be no reason for this. Obviously underlying stress, particularly in the work situation, would promote the stutter. Now you have developed and used your technique, you assume that this stress will go away, but it takes time to replace bad experiences with good ones and convince yourself that you will not stutter. Be patient.

■ COPING WITH ILLNESS

It is very difficult to keep your speech fluent when you are sick. A saving grace is that when you are sick, you are usually away from people and there is very little need to speak anyway. Of course, there are times when you feel sick and cannot afford the luxury of staying in bed and not talking. If you go to work, the very fact that you don't feel well puts your speech under pressure. In these situations try to minimise the amount of talking you do. It is very important that you do not 'soldier on' and risk giving yourself a bad bout of stuttering.

If the work you are engaged in means you cannot take time off even when you are ill, you should work out a plan of some kind to make the situation as easy as possible for yourself. I am not preaching situation avoidance here. If, because of illness (a situation beyond your control), you have lost your ability to apply your technique, it is better not to risk creating a negative experience by encountering a difficult speech situation.

Making the work situation easier

- If you are expected to attend a client meeting, explain to your manager or colleagues when you arrive at work that you are not well and have difficulty in talking. Ask them to run the meeting on this occasion and offer to attend as backup only.
- If you have been scheduled to give a presentation, do what you can to have it postponed. If this is impossible, try to find a replacement. If there is no way out of giving the presentation, explain when you stand up to speak that you have all but lost your voice. Then carry on as best you can. Use your technique as well as you can and speak as slowly as possible. Those listening will not be expecting a brilliant orator, as you have already warned them what to expect. This warning, hopefully, will also have taken some of the pressure from you, which will make it easier for you to use your technique.

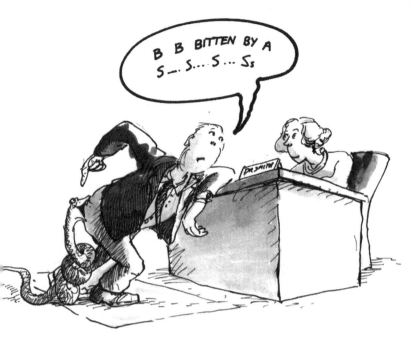

- If you have to do some telephoning at work, try to make as few calls as possible. Explain to your colleagues that your illness has affected your throat and you have difficulty speaking. Ask to be assigned non-speaking duties until you are back to normal. Every office has filing or administrative work that can be done in these circumstances.

When you are ill and you have to go into work, try to arrange for the conditions to be made as favourable as possible for you. The message here is to keep in control of the situation.

■ COPING WITH FATIGUE

Fatigue is another factor that may cause you to risk losing the grip on your technique. When you are run down you can have trouble with your speech. As with illness, try to avoid any demands for you to talk. If this is unavoidable, try to practise as much as you can to get you through whatever speaking situation you are facing.

I believe the most beneficial thing you can do when you have to speak when fatigued is to slow right down and use an obvious level of technique. You will be running close to the edge of stuttering anyway and the only way you can regain control is to use a lot of technique at a speed that makes it difficult for you to make a mistake.

Inevitably, an occasion will arise when you will have to speak, even though you are very tired. Do your best. No-one can ask more of you than that. Remember that maintaining fluency is your priority. Use your technique and slow down. You really have no choice but to talk slowly.

■ COPING WITH THOSE STUTTERY DAYS

A friend and I were once discussing how on some mornings you wake up and feel your control of your speech is shaky. My friend referred to this as 'feeling stuttery' — which I think describes it perfectly.

Stutterers will understand the term. Some days you feel really strong and think you could succeed in being fluent even in the most difficult speaking situation. Other days all you want to do is forget all about the 'fluent-speaking world'.

Speech requires physical effort. If you are feeling low physically, your speech will probably suffer. In these circumstances, the first thing you lose is control over your speech. After my clinical treatment course, I noticed that on some days I felt so good about my speech that I really did not have to work hard to keep it fluent. Other days were a disaster. I would have to do a lot of practice and generally work a lot harder on my speech and still all day I would feel 'shaky' about it.

There are steps you can take to help you through a 'feeling stuttery' day. I believe that your physical condition on the day causes you to feel stuttery. The difference between your physical well-being on a good speech day and your physical well-being on a bad speech day can be very slight, but can make a big difference to the way you speak.

The next time you wake up feeling particularly vulnerable speechwise, make a note of it in your speech diary. In particular, note what you ate during the previous day and what you had for dinner that night. Describe how you slept, whether it was sound or restless. Describe the previous day. Was it a stressful day for you? How did you speak throughout the day? Were you speaking with good technique or were you too fast and not using technique properly?

Plan of action

When you feel stuttery, you feel you have lost control over your speech and will be particularly susceptible to stuttering. To counteract this feeling of loss of control you can perform tasks that will demonstrate to yourself that you are in control of your speech. It is a fact that if you use your technique properly and slow your speech rate down, you will not stutter.

After you have got out of bed, do not talk unless you are using an obvious level of technique and are prepared to speak very slowly. I would suggest using 150 spm. Stay at this rate until you talk to your speech buddy on the phone. Tell him or her that you are feeling anxious today and are worried that you are going to stutter. Ask them to be really ruthless in their evaluation of your speech during your practice session. Try to put a lot of time into this session as it will be laying the foundation for your speech for the rest of the day. End this session at the speed you wish to maintain. Make arrangements to call your speech buddy after lunch for your second practice session.

After the first practice session and before you leave for work ensure that you are not speeding up. It is a good idea to speak at a slightly slower rate than the one you finished your practice session at. Your feeling of susceptibility to stuttering should be diminishing by now as a result of your practice session. Any areas of weakness in your technique will have been identified by and discussed with your speech buddy. You will also have the positive realisation that you have been awake for probably an hour or so on this 'feeling stuttery' day and you have spoken perfectly fluently and in perfect technique since you awoke.

The next step is really vital! You may feel that you have still not gained full control. To regain it you have to convince yourself that in order not to stutter you simply use your technique. To prove that you can do this, you need to desensitise. You must have a desensitising plan worked out to use when you get to work. I suggest you use either a voluntary stutter or an obvious level of technique with someone you would normally not feel comfortable doing this with. The purpose of this is to make you feel that you have control over your speech and not that it has control over you. The desensitising step is not an easy one to take, but it is absolutely critical if you are going to regain control of your speech. You will find that the stuttery feeling will gradually fade away. Do not forget to report back to your speech buddy!

■ COPING WITH DIFFICULT PEOPLE

We all encounter difficult people. Only the other day a person came to my office regarding some consultancy work. From the outset it was quite apparent that he was itching for an argument! It was a strange situation. He was in my office because he needed my help, yet he was confronting me at every turn. I found myself getting more and more frustrated with him, which was not helping my speech or my control over the situation generally.

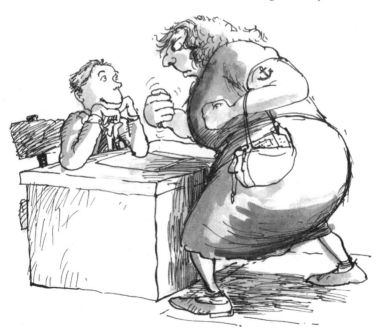

As the meeting went on I decided that the more agitated my client got, the more relaxed I would appear. I concentrated on my speed and used more and more obvious technique. I started to forget about my client's agitation and actually started to enjoy using my technique. Before treatment I would have found this situation particularly difficult and threatening, and would most certainly have stuttered. Stuttering would have made me feel that the other person had the upper hand and because of my speech I could not have argued with him. I would have let myself become vulnerable.

By using my technique I remained fluent and, more importantly, sounded calm and controlled, even though I was not. This appearance of being in control had a beneficial effect on the meeting. The person left reasonably happy. The meeting ended a lot better than it began.

RETAINING CONTROL OF THE SITUATION
When you encounter a difficult person I suggest you do the following.
1. Slow your speech down to say 180 spm. Try to maintain this rate.
2. Use a reasonably obvious level of technique. Do not worry about what the 'difficult' person may be thinking or saying.
3. If the person starts to raise their voice, lower yours. This will put you in control of the situation. The more they raise their voice, the less control of the situation they have.
4. Think before you speak. Do not say anything that you have not thought through well. Use your imaginary screen.

It is not easy to keep cool and think clearly when you are dealing with a difficult person. Although it may seem odd, in this case having a speech technique gives you an advantage. It makes you concentrate on keeping control. It makes you stay cool, think of your speech, use your technique and relax.

A FINAL WORD ON HOT SPOTS

We all have different 'hot spots' in our lives. I have recounted some of mine. I hope that you can relate your situations to mine and get benefit from my methods of dealing with them. If your hot spots are different, I am sure that you will still be able to find something of relevance in this chapter. Think carefully through my suggested approach to the situations and see how it may be used or perhaps modified to assist you in your hot spots.

No-one's perfect and I certainly am not. But I have used all the methods in this guide with success. They have all worked for me. I hope they will work for you.

CHAPTER EIGHT

WHERE DO WE GO FROM HERE?

This guide is about your stutter, how much you really want to overcome it and exactly what you intend to do to achieve fluency. Right through the guide I have spoken about speech 'technique'. I have presumed that you have a technique. If you do not I would urge you to contact speech pathologists and enquire about treatments available that may be of benefit to you.

What I have written has come from my own mind and heart. I have tried to describe all the situations that have caused me frustration and disappointment and what I have done to try and overcome stuttering. I have been successful and have enjoyed an enormous feeling of freedom as a result. It is not easy and takes a lot of work and effort; and there will still be problems. I continue to work every day at my speech and I still have the occasional problem. Compared with what I used to experience, these problems are minor. I remember when I used to come home from work totally dejected after a bad speech day. It has been three years since I have had one of those days. I want other stutterers to be able to attain this same freedom — both from the problems caused by stuttering and the feelings of dejection accompanying them.

A lot of what I have written centres around work, which I have found to be the most challenging environment. Although I describe mostly office type situations, I believe the methodology and basic messages will apply to whatever environment your situation relates to, whether it be social, professional or otherwise.

WHEN THINGS GO WRONG

As long as you can keep going and try again, there is nothing to worry about. If you stutter you are either not using technique or you are pushing yourself too hard. If it is due to an absence of technique, that's easy to fix — use your technique. If you are pushing yourself too hard, take life a little easier. Crawl before you walk.

When things go wrong for you and you feel lousy about it, get on the phone and talk to your speech buddies. That's what they are there for. Do not forget that you are not alone. Oh, and do not forget to talk to that special person in your life who would do anything for you.

Remember if you do have problems analyse what went wrong. Go back and try again.

I have devoted a whole chapter to the importance of becoming desensitised. I believe it is one of the most important messages in this guide. Stop worrying about what anyone will think of how you sound when you use obvious technique. You are dealing with your situation in a very positive way. What listeners may think is really not important. They do not stutter, you do! Desensitisation enables you to avoid reinforcing negative speaking situations. Please practise becoming desensitised. It is worth the initial embarrassment.

AN ATTAINABLE DREAM

We all have dreams of taking a pill and finding that we no longer stutter. We are fluent speakers. But when we wake, we realise there is no wizard with a magic pill. I have often dreamed of waking up fluent, but I know it is not going to happen. You know that too. The sooner you throw away the dream and start doing something constructive about controlling your speech, the sooner you will start to speak fluently.

I have enjoyed our time together and I have enjoyed getting to know you. I would like to consider you as a friend and I hope you consider me one as well. And through this book, I will always be there when you need me. Please remember that you are not alone. There are a lot of stutterers in the world and we all share the same frustrations and disappointments.

There is something else that I hope we all share and that is a sense of understanding towards people with disabilities. People who rise above their disabilities are people who really have courage and dignity. Anyone who has taken on the challenge of overcoming a disability, whatever it may be, has my lifelong admiration and respect.

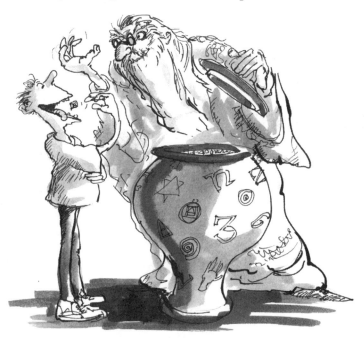

If you are really determined to stop stuttering and use your technique, you have a responsibility towards yourself whenever you speak. You have the ability to express yourself without stuttering. Use that ability. There is a lot more at stake than just speaking without stuttering. Stutterers allow themselves to live in a miserable world of fear, humiliation and denial. Stuttering prevents them from being able to speak their mind.

It is up to you to break free. Use your technique, become comfortable with it, apply it on all occasions and speak with confidence. Know that you can say what you want to, when you want to.

Fluent speech is not a dream — it can become a reality. Apply yourself, read the guide, carry it around with you and refer to it often. Consider it your mobile speech buddy — always on your side. Set your assignments, do not be too easy on yourself, but at the same time, do not be too severe a critic. The fight is worth it, not only to yourself but to others around you. You have a lot to say and we are all waiting to hear it.

FINAL TIPS FOR YOUR SURVIVAL KIT

- Try to approach speaking situations from a different point of view — see them as opportunities to improve your speech, not as something to avoid.
- Do not under any circumstances apologise if you stutter.
- You have the means as well as the right to express yourself, exercise both.
- Accept challenges — do not live in your speech comfort zone.
- Pick your speech rate and live it. It isn't easy but it does get easier.